THE DRINKING WOMAN'S DIET

WOMAN'S DIET

A Liver-Friendly Lifestyle Guide

Wendy Narby

ISBN: 978-1-4834-8611-6 (sc)
ISBN: 978-1-4834-8610-9 (e)

Library of Congress Control Number: 2018906209

Lulu Publishing Services rev. date: 06/18/2018

CONTENTS

PREFACE

THE IDEA FOR this book came about at the end of wine tour in Bordeaux. A client, groaning from a week of fabulous food and wine, asked me, "How do you do this all the time and keep in shape?" It's a comment that also comes up in my social media feed, which is dominated by pictures of wine and food. Yes, I'm one of those people.

Well, the first answer is I don't do it all the time, but I do it a lot. I drink wine for a living. I am a wine educator, wine guide, and writer with a speciality in Bordeaux.

I teach wine classes, run tastings, and talk at wine dinners around the world for professionals and enthusiastic amateurs. I take people around vineyards and wineries of Bordeaux and taste my way through other wine regions of the world. It's a wonderful job, but as with everything, there is a downside. The benefits of wine drinking may constantly be lauded in the press, but so are the risks. Adding insult to injury, wine goes with food, and tasting dinners are rarely very light affairs. Foie gras followed by duck breast anyone? So as well as keeping an eye on the state of my liver, I try to keep an eye on my waistline.

As I started sharing a few tricks and tips with my guest, she suggested I write this down and hand it out before starting the week. So the inspiration for this book started with the idea of sharing a few survival tricks and techniques—the lessons I have learned from the French, from my friends, and from therapists and other yogis to try and maintain a healthy body in what may initially appear to be an unhealthy industry.

Then a couple of things happened that made me think I should perhaps take a closer look at my drinking habits and not be too complacent (or smug) about the wine lifestyle I've chosen. At an acupuncture consultation, the therapist said, "Well, there's nothing really wrong with you, except perhaps for your liver." (He didn't know what I did for a living.) He stuck a couple of needles in between my thumb and forefinger and next to my big toes to help out. I have since learned that "liver qi stagnation" is the disorder acupuncturists say they most commonly see, so I don't feel quite so bad.

Then a few months later, I was at the Mayr Clinic in Austria; on my first consultation, the doctor looked into my eyes and pinched my cheek and said, "Aha, your liver!"

Again I hadn't even mentioned that I drink for a living. So I thought the health issues associated with booze needed a closer look.

ABOUT THE AUTHOR

I ARRIVED IN PARIS at the age of twenty, a degree in agricultural economics in my pocket and a place to study for a master's in food and wine marketing in the "City of Light." I hardly spoke a word of French.

A year later, I was fluent in French, two stone heavier, and had a job as a sales rep for a food company. It's not a glamorous as it sounds; it involved a lot of running around Paris at the crack of dawn stocking supermarket shelves. I loved every minute of it. I ate and drank everything French friends put in front of me. Friends used to joke "Il vaut mieux la voir en photo qu'à table" (It's better to see her in a photo than at your table)! After eight years in Paris, I was running the European offices for British Meat.

Wine was always on the scene—it was France of course. I was lucky, the Rotary Foundation sponsored my studies in Paris, and the local Rotary Club adopted me. One of the members owned a vineyard in Bordeaux and inspired me to write my thesis on wine marketing. A passion was born. Upon graduation, the vineyard Château de France (what a great name) asked me to represent its wines on a promotional trip to the United States. They didn't have to ask twice. It was a steep learning curve, and another vineyard owner, Hamilton Narby, graciously helped me. Eight years later, I married him and moved to Bordeaux.

Leaving Paris was a shock; thirty years ago, Bordeaux was not the vibrant and glamorous city it is today. It took a while to carve a niche for myself. I carried on commuting to Paris, consulting for previous clients, and all the while learning more about wine. I started writing about wine, finally sharing my growing passion for the region through teaching.

The chateaus in Bordeaux now welcome visitors with open arms, tables, and often guest rooms, but this wasn't the case when I starting showing clients around the region. It has been a lot of fun pioneering and sharing the emergence of wine tourism in Bordeaux and its evolution over the past twenty years.

Working in this business did nothing to shift those two stone I piled on at the beginning of my French adventure. Motherhood didn't help either. When my husband sold the vineyard and then retired, a little reassessment was needed, for both of us. Thanks to an amazing teacher, I rediscovered yoga, a passion my mother instilled into me as a teenager. This practice and the support of some wonderful girlfriends gave me the focus I needed to get healthy again. I wasn't going to stop working in the wine business, so I needed some ground rules to live by to balance the two—wine and wellness.

It is these ideas that I want to share with you in *The Drinking Woman's Diet*. At the end of some chapters, I've tried to apply the KISS (keep it simple, stupid) principles by sharing simple ideas and recommendations that should be easy to apply and to stick to.

WHY THE DRINKING WOMAN?

WELL, I'M A woman and I drink! I can only talk from my point of view and experience. As a female baby boomer, I'm right there in the category of drinkers increasing their health risks through their habits, and I'm not the only one. Many of my girlfriends are struggling with weight and fitness issues, balancing the good times with wanting to stay healthy.

Many of my friends work in the wine industry (and many, many more support it). So here are the results of my research into how to keep my liver happy and healthy while maintaining a love of wine. Let's be clear, my objective is not how to drink more but how to drink better and to understand what I can do to maintain as healthy a body as possible given my weakness. Let's face it we all have one—or two. My second one would be chocolate. Sound familiar?

I like to stay fit and healthy, and I hope to grow old not too disgracefully, but not too carefully either. My grandmother, who reached the ripe age of ninety-six, swore by a glass of Guinness everyday with lunch and a little something in her hot milk at night. My mother, at ninety-one, still takes a glass of red (Bordeaux) with lunch every day.

This book draws on advice from health and fitness specialists and information gleaned from medical reviews and books. It includes ideas that I have test-driven to help fellow wine lovers who are not prepared to give up their habit but not prepared to sacrifice their health either.

Men are of course welcome to read along, but as we'll see in chapter one, women do have an unfair disadvantage when it comes to drinking.

The recommended limits for women are lower than for men, and we'll look at the complicated relationship that women have with wine and its pitfalls, pleasures, and benefits. The effects of excess booze are seen not just in the liver but also in your eyes, in your skin, and on your waistline. If you are reading this in your bright-eyed smooth-skinned twenties, don't feel too smug—your day will come too. We will all reap the rewards of habits we cultivate now, whether good or bad.

Many of us drinking women have a sneaking feeling that we may be drinking too much. Perhaps we're piling on the pounds, not feeling too great in the morning, or just reading in the press about how much drinking is bad for us. We know that moderate drinking should be part of a healthy balanced lifestyle, including our portions of fresh fruit and veg, low sugar, no processed food, exercise, and so on and so forth. You've heard it all before. I'll look at what moderation really means and at the other lifestyle habits that can help our bodies process alcohol more efficiently and protect us from any harmful effects. I'm no paragon of virtue. I find it hard to stick to good intentions, so in chapter two when we look at the thorny question of moderation, I'll share some of the tricks I have picked up over my years (and years) in the business that help us to stick to our newfound resolutions.

These tricks are not permission to drink to excess but, rather, ways we can enjoy our allocated units and wake up fresh as a daisy the next morning.

I don't really buy into the myth that French women don't get fat; after thirty years living in France, I know that French women come in all shapes and sizes. But putting on the pounds and not being able to shift them does seem to be a problem that my Anglo-Saxon girlfriends struggle more with than do the French. French women certainly seem to drink less than their Anglo-Saxon counterparts, so in chapter four we'll look more closely at how the French drink, with some advice from my French girlfriends who also spend most of their lives in wine (in one way or another).

We'll take a brief look at wine appreciation, too. If we are drinking less, we really should drink better. I would like to share with you how to really enjoy the wine you drink, making drinking a healthy and pleasurable ritual rather than mindless overindulgence. There is more than the social pleasure of having a glass of wine with friends; there is also the pleasure of paying attention to what is in your glass.

In chapter three, we'll look at how the liver, our fabulous detox organ, works and what we can do to help it along, including some ideas for a daily detox in chapter five.

The use of the word *diet* in the title of the book may be misleading: This is not a weight-loss diet. However, by following some of these ideas, you'll be heading towards a healthier lifestyle. And if you are carrying a few extra pounds, weight loss should be a happy by-product. Not everyone who drinks is overweight; like a fine wine, it's all about balance. Rather than look at what we can't eat and drink in chapter six, we'll look at what we should include in our diet to keep us healthy.

I am a passionate yogi; wine and yoga retreats in Bordeaux are one of the ways I combine these two passions. I'm often asked how can you seriously combine wine and yoga? Aren't wine drinking and healthy living incompatible? I don't think so. Learning to pay attention to what you are drinking, being in the moment, and making the most of it sound like mindfulness, a tenet of yoga philosophy, to me. In chapter seven, we'll look at incorporating exercise, yoga or otherwise, into our lifestyles.

The strapline on my website is, "Knowledge increases pleasure." Well, knowledge is also power, power to make the right decisions. Alcohol is a subject fraught with myths, old wives' tales, and social pressures. Accurate and up-to-date information about how our bodies process alcohol, the benefits, and the potential problems is important. Research continues and the picture changes; the Internet and the press are awash with both scare stories and articles about the benefits of booze.

Deep down, you know if your drinking habit is an issue—if it's affecting your waistline, your health, your performance, and your skin.

This is not a book that will give you an excuse to drink to excess, and I'm not looking to demonise drink, either. I hope, *The Drinking Woman's Diet* will allow me to share some helpful ideas on how to enjoy wine without putting your figure, your face, your health, or your sanity at too much risk. Let's work out how to enjoy a drink and still be on top of our game.

I am not a medical practitioner. Before embarking on any major diet or exercise change, you should consult a doctor, especially if you feel your drinking is getting out of hand.

CHAPTER ONE

WOMEN AND WINE: IT'S COMPLICATED

WHAT IS ALCOHOL?

THE ALCOHOL CONTAINED in most of our favourite beverages is ethanol (ethyl alcohol). It is produced when yeast ferments sugar. It's a hydrocarbon, a mix of hydrogen, oxygen, and carbon molecules. This simple ingredient is part of a plethora of drinks. Consuming alcohol is such a pleasurable experience that we have been drinking it for thousands of years. Over time, we have created and refined the thousands of drinks that we can now choose from. We have a range of wine, beers, and spirits that defies the imagination and cataloguing. We really are spoilt for choice.

We are not all equal before alcohol, and women are even less equal. Gender is a key factor in how quickly and how well we digest alcohol. The common theory is that women are generally smaller and have less body water; the percentage of water in men's bodies helps dilute the alcohol they drink. This has an effect, but the real key is in our metabolism.

When women drink the same amount as men drink, more alcohol builds up in their bloodstreams, so those healthy-drinking limits are lower for women than for men.

Why? The enzyme alcohol dehydrogenase is responsible for breaking down alcohol.[1] It starts in the stomach, which accounts for about 20 per cent of its detoxification, but this first stage seems to work less well in women, either because we have less of the enzyme there or because oestrogens may inhibit its action. The science is still undecided. Women under forty, in particular, seem to have less of the enzyme in the stomach. As less alcohol is processed in the stomach, more passes into the small intestine, where it is absorbed directly into the blood. It then goes to the liver to be broken down. So a woman, despite drinking an equal quantity of alcohol at the same rate as a man, will have a higher BAC (blood alcohol concentration); more alcohol builds up in our bloodstreams because it is transformed more slowly. A woman's body can take one-third longer to eliminate alcohol than a man's.

As women are, as a rule, less heavy than men, this affects alcohol levels, too. (That's not an excuse to put on weight; fat doesn't work as well as muscle!) Hormones also play a role (when don't they?). Some bright-spark researcher found that women are more likely to drink in the seven days before menstruation, a finding that won't come as a surprise to any women out there.

To sum up, a sixty-kilogram woman who drinks two 175 ml glasses of 12 per cent alcohol wine over a ninety-minute period will have a BAC of 0.080 compared to just 0.037 for an eighty-kilogram man who drinks the same. More than twice as high! You can check your estimated BAC based on your drinking habits at http://www.globalrph.com/bac.cgi.

WOMEN'S DRINKING HABITS ARE DIFFERENT FROM MEN'S

Historically, fewer women than men drink, but this is changing.[2] As women become a larger part of the workforce, and in particular the executive workforce, men's drinking habits are spreading to women. This is reflected in popular culture; have you seen how much women drink on the TV series *Good Wife* and *Scandal*? The powerful leading ladies all reach for a large glass of red as soon as they walk thought the door after a hard day at the office or share a whisky with the men in times of celebration.

The role of women in the wine business has changed dramatically since I started visiting wine cellars in Bordeaux about thirty years ago. Back then, it was unusual to see a woman in a wine cellar. Now it's unusual not to. In 2007, I organised a wine tour of Bordeaux on the theme of Women in Wine. It was still a bit of a novelty then. This is no longer the case.

From cellar rats to winemakers, from managers to marketers and owners, women make up an important and influential part of the industry's workforce. The rise of the female sommelier has also done much to make the world of wine more accessible to women and to everyone, dusting off some of the fustiness so long associated with wine appreciation. It's important, as women make up the majority of wine purchasers—women purchase up to 60 per cent of wine.[3] This has come at a cost to some women's health.

Dipsomania is a nineteenth-century term for a craving for alcohol. It sounds so much more elegant than alcoholism. But whatever you want to call it, we should look at it.

Historically, when it comes to heavy drinking, women equal or surpass men in the number of problems that result. Figures from the US National Institute on Alcohol Abuse and Alcoholism (NIAAA) show female alcoholics have death rates 50 to 100 per cent higher than those of male alcoholics, including deaths from suicides, alcohol-related accidents, heart disease, stroke, and liver cirrhosis.[4]

Many women have trouble with alcohol; it can appear an easy, immediate, and everyday solution for many issues that affect us. Stress relief, anyone?

SOME WOMEN ARE MORE AT RISK OF EXCESS DRINKING THAN OTHERS

Research from the National Institute on Alcohol Abuse and Alcoholism (NIAAA) (see note 4)* suggests that a woman is more likely to drink excessively if she has any of the following:

- Blood relatives with alcohol problems
- A partner who drinks heavily
- The ability to hold her liquor better than others
- A history of depression
- A history of childhood physical or sexual abuse
- Trouble in her closest relationships

Heavy drinking is more common among single women who have never married, are living unmarried with a partner, or are divorced or separated. Why? Several things spring to mind—stress, loneliness and insecurity among them.

None of this is rocket science, but it might help you understand any issues you may have with alcohol.

THE VINTAGE EFFECT

While we're on the subject of alcohol's apparent gender discrimination, it doesn't improve with age. Ageing reduces the body's ability to adapt to alcohol; older adults reach higher blood levels of alcohol when drinking the same amount as younger people.

Why are the effects of alcohol worse after forty? (Some of us know they are.) Although younger women have less alcohol dehydrogenase enzyme, the organs that metabolise alcohol, the liver and stomach, shrink with the passing years, so more alcohol goes into the blood and stays there for longer. We become more dehydrated with age too, feeling less thirsty and drinking less water. As our bodies lose water and gain fat with the passing years (we'll be working on this later), alcohol in the blood becomes more concentrated, breaking down less quickly than it does in the bloodstream of a twenty-year-old.

If you think you become the worse for wear more quickly with the passing years and that your hangovers are worse than they used to be, you're right. It's not your imagination.

The NIAAA recommends that people aged sixty-five and older limit their consumption of alcohol to three drinks per day.[5] This sounds pretty generous. But with age, we become more discerning and can probably afford better wines than we could in our twenties.

Older women may be especially sensitive to the stigma of being alcoholic and are unlikely to admit a drinking problem. Underreporting (lying about our alcohol intake) is not something we grow out of, and alcohol problems among the elderly may be mistaken for other ageing-related conditions such as dizziness, falling, depression, or sleeping problems, to name a few. This situation can lead healthcare providers to miss or fail to treat alcohol problems in older women.

It is also worth noting that some of the signs of diabetes—dizziness, disorientation, and sleepiness—are similar to drunkenness. They may be written off as the result of a few too many drinks when, in fact, they may be a sign of something more serious. Diabetics are particularly at risk from excess alcohol, especially when drinking on an empty stomach. Beware if you are or may be diabetic, and don't dismiss low blood sugar symptoms as drunkenness. If you haven't been drinking or have hardly drunk at all and are experiencing these symptoms, get yourself checked for diabetes.

CANCER

Cancer has come to the centre of the alcohol debate. The World Health Organization has classified alcohol as a known carcinogen. On its list, alcohol comes after tobacco, obesity, other dietary factors, and lack of exercise. According to the charity Drinkaware, more than one-fifth of alcohol-related deaths are due to cancer, which is a lot fewer than violent or accidental deaths but is still significant.[6] Chronic drinking may increase your risk of developing certain cancers, including cancers of the mouth, oesophagus, throat, and liver, as well as, in certain cases, breast and even colon or rectal cancer. Why? As our bodies process alcohol, it is broken down into acetaldehyde and then into acetic acid. Acetaldehyde is a highly reactive and toxic by-product that, in excess, may contribute to tissue breakdown, forming damaging molecules that may cause genetic mutations favouring certain cancers.

For a sixty-year-old woman, the benefit/risk calculations for alcohol consumption are tricky.

Although breast cancer is one of the cancers most often associated with alcohol consumption in women, postmenopausal women may benefit from alcohol's cardiovascular protective effects; it's worth bearing in mind that, in the United Kingdom, ten times more women die each year from heart disease than from breast cancer. Women tend to be more afraid of developing breast cancer than heart disease, as it is a much more emotive subject. Women with a family history of breast cancer or who use hormone replacement therapy (HRT) may be particularly at risk, as alcohol can increase the amounts of some hormones in the body, including oestrogen, that certain types of breast cancer are sensitive to.

OUR COMPLEXION

Complexion is another subject close to our hearts. Heavy alcohol consumption can reduce vitamin A levels, which are really important for healthy and elastic skin; vitamin A helps collagen and elastin production.[7] It's not just inhibitions that alcohol loosens! The way the liver processes vitamin A from the food we eat, into a form that the body can use is similar to how it processes alcohol. With an excess of alcohol, the liver struggles to multitask and produce enough of vitamin A.

Alcohol can also increase flushing; this does not affect everyone but can be really embarrassing for sufferers. People with less of the enzymes needed to break down alcohol become red-faced very quickly when tasting even small amounts of wine. But long-term excess drinking can lead to blood vessels becoming enlarged, leaving permanent redness and broken blood vessels for anyone. Alcoholics are often represented in cartoons as having a big red nose. Not a good look, ladies. Alcohol is a diuretic; it causes the body to lose water, which contributes to dry skin, leading to that dried-out look that smokers and drinkers often have. Alcohol can also affect digestion and may lead to leaky gut syndrome, which has been linked to acne rosacea.

BRAINWORK

Researchers found that the negative effects on cognitive function were more serious in male chronic or binge drinkers than women, possibly due to the protective effect of oestrogen.[8] Oestrogen may also go some way to protecting women from the permanent brain damage that can be caused by alcohol.

Don't be complacent. In moderation, alcohol is unlikely to kill your brain cells, but heavy drinking—see the moderation chapter below for safe recommendations—will. Peripheral nerves are affected too (alcoholic neuropathy). This damage is not due to dying cells; brain cell shrinkage and impaired communication between brain cells can cause cognitive problems.

The good news is that this alcohol-induced deterioration will stop when the person stops drinking; some recovering alcoholics regain brain volume from both supportive cells and the partial return of existing neurons to normal size. However, once neurons die, they are gone.[9]

BONE STRENGTH

Excess drinking reduces bone density, affecting the uptake of calcium and vitamin A from the stomach and their metabolism by the pancreas and liver. This is especially important in younger women, as bone mass builds up to the age of thirty-five. It is very important that young women who do drink to excess preserve their future bones. However, there is some proof that moderate drinking may help increase bone strength in postmenopausal women, due to the effect on oestrogen.[10] However, moderation is key. Nice to know there's some advantage to getting older. But beware! If you're blasted, you're more likely to fall over, which will not help keep your bones intact.

MOOD SWINGS

Blood sugar spikes with alcohol consumption, increasing insulin production, transforming any sugar in the blood, and resulting in very low blood sugar. This makes you feel tired, hungry, and irritable. Sound familiar? Have you ever bitten someone's head off after a few drinks? It's the combination of low blood sugar putting you in a bad mood, reduced inhibitions, and reduced self-control. It's not necessarily a personality disorder or PMT!

THAT TIME OF LIFE: ALCOHOL AND MENOPAUSE

The liver tends to kick in at about 4 a.m. and functions at a higher temperature than the rest of the body. When it's busy eliminating alcohol and other toxins, it produces a lot of heat, which really doesn't help if you are struggling with hot nights. Have you ever woken hot and sweaty at about 4 a.m.? If so, you are not alone; you have no idea how many people look wide-eyed at me when I suggest this. It may be due to a certain time of life, but try not to eat or drink heavily late at night for a few weeks, and see if it makes a difference. You'll probably find it will help with those heart palpitations we associate with the change of life, too.

SAFE DRINKING FOR WOMEN

Aside from health issues associated with excess alcohol, there are also social consequences. I'm not being sexist here; the sorry spectacle of a drunken man has equally as little charm in my eyes as that of a drunken woman. However, according to the World Health Organisation (WHO), heavy drinking (by both men and women) does increase a woman's risk of becoming a victim of violence.[11]

Being tipsy may make you feel erudite and like a dancing queen, but we all really know the true story. Now, with smart phones and social media, so, unfortunately, does everyone else! Nobody is perfect, and getting drunk happens. Outrageous dancing is one thing. But young people, especially young women, are particularly at risk from heaving drinking. Aside from the effects on their health and their brains, particularly damaging on a younger brain, these risks include violence (including sexual violence) from others and self-inflicted, accidents, and sexually transmitted disease from unprotected sex. Alcohol lowers inhibitions, leading to rash decisions we may regret the next day. Booty calls and drunk-dialling, anyone?

Don't put yourself or your friends at risk. Look out for your girlfriends when out partying (that goes for men as well as women) and stay together. Always have a designated driver. It's also an good idea to have designated carer, even if no one is driving, who stays sober enough look out for the team, making sure everyone gets home safely.

ALCOHOL POISONING

Alcohol poisoning is life threatening. Symptoms include:

- Confusion and stupor
- Vomiting
- Seizures
- Slow, irregular breathing
- Low body temperature and bluish skin

If you see someone vomit several times or pass out after drinking heavily, there is a risk of severe dehydration or even brain damage. Get medical help immediately.

THE DARK SIDE

As if weight gain, bad skin, red noses, and a hangover weren't ugly enough, there is a very ugly and dark side to alcohol abuse. Violence, accidents, mental heath problems, crime, and absenteeism are a few of the issues associated with excess alcohol. Alcohol abuse costs up to £21 billion a year to the health services in England alone. Young people are particularly at risk; excess alcohol consumption among young adults is associated with a higher risk of traumatic injury and death than in middle-aged and older drinkers. Middle-aged women drinkers are at lower risk; there has to be some advantage to growing older (and wiser perhaps?).

LET'S TALK ABOUT SEX

The first sip of booze can act as a social lubricant; we feel a slight buzz, more open and more relaxed. Terms like "Dutch courage" describe how we feel more confident about taking a risk—able to approach that attractive person across the room. You may feel sexier, but that glass of wine may also make you look sexier: A Bristol University study showed that drinking dilated the pupils and relaxed the facial muscles, making people look more attractive.[12] You might even flush a little, which is also charming. Beware—this works but only up to one glass. After that, things might start to get a little more ugly.

"Beer goggles" is a rather unattractive term to describe a loosening of sexual inhibitions and discretion in approaching potential partners. It's usually used as a joke to explain why you flirted with someone you would not normally have found attractive. The more scientific term is alcohol myopia theory (AMT). Inebriated people tend to concentrate on the sexual attractiveness cues and sweep aside normal inhibitors, giving in to urges that they might otherwise resist.

A little alcohol might act as an aphrodisiac, reducing inhibitions, and it can even increase sexual arousal, but it doesn't always mean you can follow through. Studies show that sexual behaviour in women under the influence of alcohol is different from that of men.[13] Well, we knew that! The effects of alcohol are balanced between its suppressive effects on sexual physiology, decreasing sexual activity, and its suppression of psychological inhibitions, increasing desire. Decisions, decisions.

Another sobering thought—high alcohol and vigorous sex both lower blood sugar, and combining the two (it happens) could cause a dangerous low. You have been warned!

Alcohol can also reduce sperm count in men. It may reduce fertility in women too; women starting IVF are often encouraged to stop drinking before treatment.

While a drink may put us in the mood for love,[14] according to a 2004 study, tipsy women needed much more stimulation to have an orgasm than did women who had little or nothing to drink, and that orgasm was less intense.[15] Some women report feeling more pleasure subjectively, which may be thanks to that relaxed feelings after their first drink. Drink too much, and dizziness, nausea, and even depression might set in. Not very sexy.

Sexual arousal needs a certain volume of blood to bring oxygen and greater sensation to the genitals. We know this is the case with the male erection, but it works for women too. Alcohol may be a vaginal lubricant as well as a social one! Increasing blood flow to the genitals is one thing, but the dehydration common when drinking too much alcohol can contribute to fatigue, headaches, and vaginal dryness. Not quite so sexy. Exchange that extra glass of wine for water to combat the effects of dehydration. Choose your drink wisely. Alcohol in moderation might help with sexual pleasure and desire, but it seems red wine has a particular effect on sex drive in women.

Research by Italians in Chianti (where else?) showed that red wine specifically increased blood flow to women's erogenous areas, which in turn led to increased levels of desire. [16] Sexual desire is linked to the presence of testosterone in men and in women. Quercetin, a polyphenol in red wine, blocks the enzyme that helps excrete testosterone. The researchers were quick to point out that, after more than a drink or two, other effects of alcohol led to a less pleasurable experience, lowering testosterone and decreasing the sex drive in men, as alcohol metabolism reduces the enzymes needed for testosterone production.

So in the interests of your sex appeal, performance, and enjoyment, it's the same old story—moderation. A light level of alcohol intake is when we're most likely to perform at our best, so don't overdo it and miss that window of opportunity!

If moderate wine consumption will keep our hearts and our sex life healthy, what exactly is moderation? Read on.

THE KISS PRINCIPLES FOR DRINKING WOMEN

- Women cannot safely drink as much as men. Get used to it.
- Heavy drinking is even more dangerous for younger women but much more painful for older woman.
- Take time to assess your drinking habits.
- Always stay safe when drinking. There's a fine line between carefree and reckless.

CHAPTER TWO

MODERATION, MOTIVATION, AND MINDFULNESS

Everything in moderation, including moderation.
—Oscar Wilde

MODERATION

BEFORE WE START looking at a diet to help us towards a healthy liver, we really do need to look at how much we are really drinking. You can eat as healthily as you like and exercise as much as you like, but too much alcohol will always take its toll. So how much is too much? Most research seems to conclude that moderate alcohol consumption, particularly red wine, may have health benefits, thanks to the polyphenols extracted from grape skins. What does moderate really mean and how can we leverage the motivation we need to be moderate in a world of temptation?

There is no one hard and fast rule for safe levels of alcohol consumption (shame, I work well to a rule book). While levels differ from person to person, everyone metabolises (breaks down) alcohol differently, resulting in dramatic differences in its absorption into the bloodstream. Our genes, largely, decide on the type and concentration of enzymes in our livers, and this dictates the rate of alcohol breakdown, our reaction to alcohol, and the resulting by-products. This is why some people flush, while others get tipsy quickly or are more or less susceptible to alcoholism and liver disease. Blood alcohol concentration (BAC) determines alcohol's effect on the body. The quicker alcohol is metabolised, the less stays in the bloodstream, the lower BAC, and the lower the risk of adverse effects and intoxication.

It's not just your genes. Your gender and your age are important but the three primary things that influence the rate at which alcohol is metabolised and, thus, BAC are:

- The alcoholic strength of what you drink
- Your drinking habits
- Your eating habits

The question sounds obvious, but how strong is that drink? You might think that an extra degree or two of alcohol on the wine label would not make that much difference. It's wine, right? Did you even know different wines have different alcohol levels? Most white wines tend to fall between 12 per cent and 14 per cent, while reds are between 13 per cent and 14.5 per cent. Read the labels. They vary enormously—from about 10 per cent for a German Riesling to over 15 per cent for a Napa Cabernet or Australian Shiraz, among many others.

All booze for sale must legally mention the alcohol level on the label, but legislation varies from country to country. In the United Kingdom, alcoholic beverages are measured in ABV (alcohol by volume) as a percentage. Thus, 10 per cent ABV (you may see "10% vol." or "10°") means that there are ten volumetric units of pure ethanol in one hundred equal units of the drink.

In the United States, labelling is different. The term "proof" is often used. Proof is about twice the ABV, so 10 per cent ABV equals about 20 proof. Likewise, 100 proof does not mean pure alcohol but 50 per cent ABV. It's still a pretty strong drink.

How accurate a measure is it? EU regulations permit a tolerance of plus or minus 0.5 per cent; looser US regulations allow a tolerance of plus or minus 1.5 per cent of alcohol for wines under 14 per cent alcohol, and plus or minus 1 per cent for wines over 14 per cent. A US wine label of 13.5 per cent could contain 15 per cent alcohol.

Alcohol levels can make a big difference. A 13 per cent and a 15 per cent alcohol by volume might not sound very different, but the effect on BAC is. While 2 per cent sounds small, it is about a 20 per cent jump in alcohol level, and blood alcohol levels can rise up 33 per cent to 43 per cent, depending on gender, on such a seemingly small difference.

HOW OFTEN?

You might be surprised to know regular drinking of moderate amounts is better for you than being virtuous all week and overdoing it at the weekend. The liver produces the enzymes responsible for breaking down alcohol as and when they are needed; drinking one or two glasses of wine daily keeps the liver stimulated to make more of this alcohol dehydrogenase enzyme. People who drink daily are capable of metabolising more alcohol than those who drink only on the weekends, as their livers contain more of the enzyme. After consuming the same amount of alcohol, a regular drinker will have a lower BAC than the sporadic drinker. This doesn't mean that regular drinking during the week gives you the right to binge drink on the weekend. The poor liver can never induce enough enzymes to offset the potentially lethal effects of binge-drinking, which is always hazardous.

Those of you who claim never to get a hangover, I hope it's because you are drinking moderately as well as regularly. If you are drinking regularly and heavily and still not getting a hangover, it is not a good sign! Tolerance is a physiological response; the more you consume, the more your body needs to have the same effect. As the levels of these enzymes in the liver increase, your tolerance builds, and you need more alcohol to get the same effects. Brains get tolerant to alcohol too. If you can still walk in a straight line after drinking a lot, it means your brain has adapted. Here starts the descent into alcoholism. The next day, the brain cells are expecting alcohol, and withdrawal symptoms such as anxiety and jitteriness can occur. You can find yourself reaching for a drink to alleviate these symptoms.

Breaking your drinking cycle is an important way to test for—and tackle—this kind of dependence. Taking a few days off can help to "reset" your tolerance level.

KEEPING THE BAC AT BAY

There's no magic way to reduce BAC, except drinking less. Drinking water does help but mainly because it slows down the speed of your alcohol intake (you drink less quickly if you intersperse each glass of wine with a glass of water). It doesn't really dilute the alcohol, as your kidneys will only allow so much water into your system. A normal liver will break down alcohol at a rate of about eight grams (one unit) per hour. Time is a great healer!

Eating helps to slow down BAC, and other factors include our general health, our body mass, and our fat to muscle ratios. Fitter healthier bodies break down alcohol more efficiently.

CURRENT RECOMMENDATIONS

Working out safe levels of wine (or any alcohol) consumption is a minefield. Some experts don't think there is any safe level and that alcohol is a poison that affects the liver, serves as a trigger for certain cancers, and is a factor affecting other health issues. And that's before we even touch on the social problems of alcohol abuse.

Then again, there is constant argument that moderate consumption of alcohol (as well as other ingredients, in wine in particular) can be health enhancing. Recommended levels of alcohol consumption vary and depend on which website or authority you consult.

THE UK GUIDELINES

Guidelines in the United Kingdom, issued by the British National Health Service, have recently been reassessed down to 14 units of alcohol for men and women, spread over one week.[17] A small glass of wine (125 ml) is considered 1.6 units so that's just less than nine small glasses of wine per week or one and a third bottles. (Am I sounding desperate yet?) Over the week is the key. Binge-drinking your whole allowance on Friday night is not part of the plan. They also recommend a couple of booze free days a week.

This is also what the British Liver Trust recommends.[18] Their "Love your Liver Campaign" reiterates the same advice, including the idea of giving your liver a couple of days off a week by not drinking alcohol. It also has a self-assessment liver health page. But to get any advantage from it, you have to tell the truth!

THE US GUIDELINES

Guidelines in the United States are about the same but more sexist, giving men the green light to drink double the allowance of women—one drink per day for women and two for men. [19] What constitutes "a drink" is also fairly fluid (excuse the pun). In wine terms here, one drink is defined as five fluid ounces of wine (12 per cent alcohol), which is about 150 ml, almost a bottle and a half a week. It also depends on what you drink; spirits have a higher level, and most beers have a lower number of units per serving than wine. It's worth checking the level of some craft beers though.

ARE YOU A BINGE DRINKER?

We all have seen photos of young people drinking to excess at the weekend. This is what we associate with binge-drinking. The trend of preloading—drinking volumes of affordable booze at home before arriving to party in bars and clubs, where prices are high, has contributed to this. It's not just young people. The Global Drug Survey in the United Kingdom found that well over half of women and around three-quarters of men drink at "levels associated with harm."[20] Data from a Sheffield University study found that it is mid-lifers, not students, who are the most prone to "preloading" (in France, we call this the rather more attractive "aperitif"), regularly enjoying 14 units of alcohol in an evening, a woman's weekly limit, according to the NHS.[21] A study of 9,000 over-fifties found they were more likely than any other age group to drink to "harmful" levels. Wisdom with age? Perhaps not. Hard drinking is dangerous at any age; it leads to higher risk of hypertension, diabetes, heart disease, stroke, and death following a heart attack.

It's not all bad news. According to the United Kingdom's Office of National Statistics, binge-drinking rates among young people are sharply down, from 29 per cent in 2005 to 18 per cent in 2013.[22] In the United States, underage drinking dropped by one-fifth between 2002 and 2013, with an estimated quarter of sixteen- to twenty-four-year-olds now teetotal, a proportion that went up by more than 40 per cent from 2006 to 2013. This is good news, as excess drinking can affect younger people in the longer term more severely than older people.

SO HOW MUCH DO YOU REALLY DRINK?

Being brutally honest with yourself about your alcohol consumption is hard. Doctors always say patients lie about their alcohol intake (more politely known as under-reporting). It's not your doctor you are lying to but yourself.

DO YOU THINK YOU HAVE A PROBLEM?

The CAGE questionnaire is a good place to start.[23] Ask yourself these questions:

- **C** Have you ever felt you should *cut down* on your drinking?
- **A** Have people *annoyed* you by criticising your drinking?
- **G** Have you ever felt bad or *guilty* about your drinking?
- **E** *Eye-opener*: Have you ever had a drink first thing in the morning to steady your nerves or to get rid of a hangover?

Two yeses merit a rethink.

There is also a more detailed questionnaire online—the Alcohol Use Disorders Identification Test (AUDIT).[24]

YOUR LIFE, YOUR BODY, YOUR HEALTH: TAKE CHARGE

The recommended levels of consumption mentioned above would appear to pose few health risks for most adults who choose to drink and who do so in a sensible manner as part of a healthy diet and lifestyle. A little of what we fancy may well do us good, but too much can be an unmitigated disaster.

Many women have trouble with alcohol. Being aware of your drinking habits is important. Understanding when and why you drink is key. Creating this awareness around your drinking habits allows you to make conscious decisions about what, when, and where to drink. It's not always easy, but it's very empowering.

If you are, or someone you know is, suffering abuse at the hands of someone with an alcohol problem, help is available. See resources at the end of the book for more information.

SO HOW MUCH SHOULD YOU BE DRINKING?

I try and work to no more than two glasses of wine a day (this can be replaced by a whisky, G&T or other cocktails as preferred). It's also important to take no fewer than two days off drinking each week.

We'll look at this healthy lifestyle. But I can hear you crying out. How on earth am I going to stick to these recommended levels? Two small glasses a day? You're kidding!

MOTIVATION

The first thing is to understand our motivation for picking up a glass; the second is to make every single one of those units count!

Let's take a look at our drinking habits and make a conscious decision to raise that glass, rather than doing so because "it's what I usually do about here and about now".

What is going through your mind when you reach for that glass of wine? Many women have a troubled relationship with alcohol. Creating awareness around your drinking habits and making those conscious decisions when it comes to what, when, and where to drink is very empowering. It's a muscle. Use it or lose it. And once you start taking control and deciding exactly when, what, and how you want to drink, the enjoyment when you choose to drink the good stuff in a good place will only be heightened. A little diligence and self-care go a long way.

Denial is often a core aspect of addiction. I do not deal with severe alcohol addiction, as it is beyond the scope of this book. But help is at hand if you feel you need it.[25]

I DRINK FOR A LIVING. WHAT'S YOUR EXCUSE?

> *Why the drink? Consider whether any of the following motivations for drinking apply to you:*

- Is it boredom, stress, depression? Or perhaps nothing is going through your mind. Is drinking just a reflex? Perhaps you're thirsty?

- Are you giving yourself a reward? I deserve a drink after the day I've had. Well done for getting that job done. I'll have a drink to celebrate.
- Is it a tonic to combat exhaustion? I'll just have a drink to pick myself up and get myself going.
- Is it punctuation? It's the end of the working day. I'm just getting home. I'm putting on the dinner. The kids are in bed. It's wine o'clock.
- Is it social lubrication? Alcohol can act as tranquiliser for stressed or nervous people, especially in a social situation.
- Are you drinking to lift your spirits? Research shows we experience pleasure when drinking alcohol, as it releases endorphins in the brain regions associated with pleasure and rewards.[26] It also increases the release of dopamine, which triggers satisfaction. These good feelings can be addictive, encouraging us to reach for a drink. Depression is closely linked to heavy drinking in women. Here lies dangerous territory; it is both cause and effect. Drinking your way out of depression, whether it's just a cheer up when you're not feeling great or turning to the bottle in severe depression, is a recipe for disaster, as alcohol exacerbates depression.
- Is it stress? Stress seems to be a common theme in women's lives. It's not clear just how stress may lead to problem drinking, but heavy drinking can lead to more stress, both professionally and personally. It's a vicious circle. There is a condition known as "Hurried Woman Syndrome." If you suffer from this, you won't need me to explain, but it's good to know there's a phrase for it and you're not alone. There's even a book about it by American gynaecologist Dr Brent Bost.[27] Often brought on by a busy lifestyle, as well as family pressure, this stress may start to feel "normal" but can have long-term consequences for the woman concerned and for those around her.
- Are you using alcohol as self-medication? Alcohol has always been used to relieve pain. Laboratory studies confirm that alcohol reduces pain, and recent research suggests that as many as 28 per cent of people experiencing chronic pain turn to alcohol to alleviate their suffering.[28]

A glass of wine marks the moment you award
yourself a unit of pleasure. Sheer joy.
— Clare Convile, *The Book for Dangerous Women*[29]

Where do these habits come from?

Using alcohol to relax may be something you have picked from family, friends, or colleagues. Or it may even be something you've seen on TV. Do you expect alcohol to remove your stress? If that's what people in your past or present do, it's hard to be different—until you start.

Any control freaks out there? Surely not! This is one occasion when your inner control freak can come into her own. Self-restraint and delayed gratification are good habits to get into. Great muscles to flex and cultivate.

Knowing that there are downsides to excess drinking, many of them cosmetic (expanding waistline, red noses, dry skin anyone?) may be the motivation we need to get a grip on how to drink with moderation. With an informed approach to drinking, we'll be slimmer with glowing skin, bright-eyed and bushy-tailed, and still a fun girl at the party as we sip on our chosen beverage.

HABITS ARE IMPORTANT

It's not so easy to change ingrained habits, but we can reprogramme ourselves. In her excellent book *The Willpower Instinct*, Dr Kelly McGonigal explains "how self control works, why it matters, and what you can do to get more of it".[30] One of the wonderful things about the book is it removes the self-loathing that many women have for not having enough self-control. If this sounds familiar, I highly recommend you read her book. According to McGonigal, willpower is a muscle, but like other muscles, it can get tired. You may be using it for all sorts of things—what to eat (or not to eat), your exercise regime, holding your tongue at home or at work, finishing a job you don't want to do. In fact, you may be using it so much that, by the end of the day, you have used up all the energy in that muscle and just have none left to resist that glass of rosé.

McGonigal states that guilt, stress, and shame don't work as motivators. So we can stop all that right away then—great news! It's all about self-acceptance and paying attention and being in the moment and making deliberate choices, rather than running on autopilot. The secret is creating new habits, good ones. Once something becomes a habit, you won't waste any valuable willpower on decision-making. You'll just do it. These habits aren't just about drinking. They apply to anything you struggle with and beat yourself up about, exhausting that willpower muscle. Twenty-one days is the time it takes to create a new habit pathway in the brain, whether it's drinking less alcohol, drinking more water, or taking more exercise. The secret is to do it little by little, with a little help.

SET SOME GOALS OR SOME GROUND RULES

I love goals. I find having clear goals, rather than a vague "Yeah, I'm cutting back," helps in realising your objectives. Make your goals positive. A "don't" at the beginning of a phrase makes us immediately want to do whatever follows, contrary lot that we are. So instead of "Don't drink alone," write, "Drink with friends."

Find some goals that work for you. Here are some I try and stick to:

- Two drinks a day
- Two days off booze a week
- Drink in company
- Drink at lunch or in the evening
- Drink two litres of water a day
- Only drink alcohol if you find it delicious

Goals should be SMART

SMART goals are specific, measurable, attainable, relevant, and time-bound. For example, drink two glasses a day.

I'm beginning to sound like a classic self-help book. (I love them, by the way. There's a few mentioned in the notes at the end of the book!) Setting precise goals, writing them down, and envisaging sticking to them really works. And we need all the help we can get here. What harm can it do?

Write your goals down. Then see yourself sticking to them. Imagine the person you will become once you do stick to them (slim, fit, healthy, sleeping better—whatever your motivation for cutting back is). Like this new you, your future self. Don't hate her for being perfect! This will help.

This is particularly important if you are heading out for an event where you know you will be challenged. Visualise yourself only drinking a small amount of lovely wine and enjoying it, saying no to a fill-up before you are ready, engaging in interesting conversation, and putting the glass down between drinks rather than desperately clinging on to it—you know your triggers. You can even concentrate on laughing (inwardly) at all the drinkers making fools of themselves. Harsh, I know, but whatever it takes!

If you didn't stick to all your goals, don't beat yourself up when you get home. Congratulate yourself for trying and for any small victories you made (I drank water first, I said no twice, I ate before drinking). Good on you.

Rules may be for fools, but having a framework within which you plan your drinking does help. Call them rules or goals or objectives—whatever floats your boat. Even if you break them, having a framework within in which you operate will help with accountability and will allow you to take stock of how, when, where, and why you are drinking.

These ground rules have to be ones that work for you. Only you know how to get the most enjoyment out of your allocation.

WHEN DO YOU DRINK?

Setting time parameters for drinking is a good way to manage moderation. Wine o'clock, the sun going down behind the yardarm, it must be 6 p.m. somewhere—phrases that show we are aware the drinking shouldn't start before a certain hour. Sundowners? Tricky in midwinter when the sun goes down at 4.30 p.m. That's a long evening of drinking ahead!

Sometimes that drink at the end of the day might be about a slight and welcome relinquishing of control or your need to unwind. Just be aware of what you are doing. You can make having a drink a decision, not a reflex.

There's nothing more desperate than watching the clock and grabbing the bottle at 6 p.m. on the dot. If this sounds familiar, you may need more help than this book can give you.

DELAYED GRATIFICATION

Delaying gratification is not a very modern concept—these days are all about right here, right now—but it's a wonderful thing to cultivate. McGonigal (mentioned above) explains that very young children who practise delayed gratification go on to be the most successful human beings, socially and financially.[31] Deferring gratification is a marker of positive adult behaviour, but it also intensifies pleasure.

Want a drink? Wait ten minutes, just ten minutes; take away the impulse. This ten-minute rule works for doing things as well as for not doing things— stopping procrastination, sticking to an exercise regime, overspending, to name a few. It gets quite exciting and empowering once you start. Often, in ten minutes, the urge has gone. The later you start, the less you will drink. Plus, once we have a drink inside us, we are more relaxed and less inclined to exercise willpower. Starting later is easier than stopping when you are on a roll.

Think about when exactly wine time or wine o'clock comes around in your household/office/life. Is it when you or your partner walk through the door at the end of the working day and kick off your shoes? "Oh, it's great to be home. I need a drink." Do you reach for the wine bottle when the kids are finally in bed (or do you need a glass to get through the bedtime routine)? Do you call in at a bar with work colleagues on the way home? I tend to reach for a glass when I'm cooking dinner. Wine goes with food goes with wine, right?

Try these ideas to implement the *ten-minute rule*:

- Start with a glass of water. This pushes back the start of drinking, slows down your consumption, and gives you something else to do with your hands if you are in a social situation where you are nervous (or bored). See above.
- Have a cup of tea. Really, if you are reaching for the wine bottle to refresh your flagging body and/or soul, a quick cuppa does the job. Of course I am English, which might explain why this works for me! A cup of tea will rehydrate, it has as many polyphenols as wine, and you won't feel like a drink straight away afterwards. Job done. This works for the boredom, procrastination, and thirst triggers, too.
- Take some exercise. Go for a walk. You'll be slimmer and drink less.
- Schedule a workout right before you expect to drink. Afterwards, you'll want to reach for something refreshing and hydrating, like water or coconut water—not something dehydrating, like alcohol.
- Or schedule an early morning workout. Knowing you have to get up and exercise in the morning is a great motivator for not drinking too much the night before. You know how much it will hurt. Make sure you have an accountability partner the next morning, someone you don't want to let down.
- Breathe. This slows down your heart rate, relaxes you, and gives you time to think and to hang on for another ten minutes.

- Check Facebook. Ha! How many times does a self-help book tell you to do that? This doesn't work if your FB feed is full of pictures of what your friends are drinking (Like mine).
- Phone a friend. Drinking on the phone still counts as drinking alone!
- Take a bath. If you are reaching for a glass to relax, this works. Throw in some Epsom salts and detox at the same time.
- Clean your teeth. Carry mints or breath strips. A minty mouth cuts the craving for just about everything alcoholic and wine in particular.
- Put your feet up and read a chapter of a book—without a glass in your hand.

STICKING TO IT

Get your friends on board. Drinking less in company is tricky; standing out from the crowd is not easy. Peer pressure is a powerful thing, and cutting back is even more difficult if friends or partners are saying, "Go on, just have another one." (The same goes for dessert when you are trying to cut back on sugar.) Good friends should be supportive; however, this lack of support might not be about you. You cutting back might shine a light on a friend's own issues with drinking. It's not always an easy subject to broach.

Choose your friends as carefully as you choose your wine. We become the people we surround ourselves with, and willpower is contagious. Avoid friends who are simply looking for a drinking partner. Getting friends on board and, even better, as accountability partners will be a huge help. This works for everything, not just controlling booze intake. I would be lost without the support of my girlfriends.

Little white lies can be a way of resisting peer pressure, such as, "I'm on antibiotics," or, "I have a hangover from last night." As a last resort, you can also say "I'm watching my weight" (not necessarily a lie). Some friends may relate to this more easily than to controlling units. If they say, "You don't need to lose weight," just answer, "Well, exactly. Limiting my booze is why!"

Those of us who work in the wine business have the advantage of being able to taste and then spit out—not exactly a polite social habit or correct dinner party behaviour.

DRINK BEFORE YOU DRINK

Always drink a glass of water before your beverage. I can't stress this enough. It slakes thirst, helps reduce dehydration and hangovers, stops you gulping your drink, pushes back the start time, etc. If you take one thing away from this book, this would be it.

I battle with drinking enough water (see chapter five). Often the first glass of wine, especially champagne, white wine, or even a G&T of an evening will slip down, hardly touching the sides. I now try and remember to ask for a drink of water first—and then hang onto the water glass, so I can sip water in between drinks.

DRINKING ALONE

It can be a pretty sad image, but it's a very pervasive one. All those TV series show women arriving back home, immediately opening a bottle, and knocking it back. Not drinking alone is a good rule (let's make that positive—drink in company). It's also a rule I break frequently, especially when a delicious drop is left in a bottle from the night before. I'll make myself a lovely lunch and sit there and really enjoy glass of wine I've chosen to go with it. That doesn't sound too sad, does it?

CHOOSE YOUR GLASSES WITH CARE

I'm not referring to the glasses on your nose, although it helps if you can see what you are drinking (see p 29). Rather, I'm referring to the glasses you are drinking out of. Size matters. Have you noticed how big the wine glasses are in bars and restaurants now? When you ask for a glass of wine, you get a goblet. Professional wisdom may be that bigger glasses allow us to swirl and sniff and perhaps show that you take your wine seriously. "Just look at these wonderful wine glasses I am serving the wine in." Honestly, some of them feel as if you could just dive in there. Research at Cambridge University showed that larger glasses make you drink more.[32] (They need research for that, really?) Even experienced bartenders will pour more alcohol into a short wide glass than a tall thin one if not using a measure.

I have a similar issue about coffee cups that look more like soup bowls, but that's probably because I've been drinking espresso in France for too long.

We (or rather I) have set us a goal of two glasses a day, five days a week, which sounds reasonable. But do check how big that glass is. It depends how attentive your waiter or barman is, too. Wine lists by the glass usually offer a range of small or large glasses. The small are rarely that small and the large, often 250 ml, represent one-third of a bottle, in which case, depending on the alcohol level, a single glass could be half your weekly allowance all in one go. Whoops! We can think it's just one glass regardless of the size and come back for more quickly, drinking more than we would if we had two "small" glasses of 125 ml instead of one of 250 ml.

YOU DON'T HAVE TO ORDER A BOTTLE

Drinking wine by the glass (see above) has never been easier. The range of wines on offer, not only in restaurants and wine bars, but also by the glass has increased, along with the range of glassware. If your local is still serving ghastly vinegar as an excuse for wine, don't waste your units there. Drink something else and save them for something lovely. It might even make the local up its game. Ask when the bottle was opened. If the wine you've been served is oxidised, send it back. We are talking our precious units here—don't waste them!

ARE YOU BEING SERVED?

It is easier when purchasing wine by the glass to keep track of consumption. When sharing a bottle with friends, your glass is likely to be topped up, regularly, so you need to keep a beady eye on just how often this is done.

Try to finish your glass before allowing a refill—not always that easy when it comes to generous hosts, you can always say I'm going to change to red next—if there's a choice on offer.

Just because someone poured you a glass doesn't mean you have to finish it. This is more important than manners. You wouldn't finish reading a book if you didn't enjoy the first few chapters or watch a film to the end you're not enjoying, would you? If you do order a bottle, you don't have to finish it, either. Just saying.

WATER IT DOWN

Worried that it's sacrilege to water down wine? Don't be. Many wine insiders drink spritzers. Use mineral water, not lemonade—too much sugar. Don't hesitate to water down your drinks with ice cubes either. The grand champagne houses are now bringing out slightly sweeter cuvées, designed especially for the "piscine" or swimming pool—champagne served in large glasses over ice cubes. The wine world can be perceived as stuffy and intimidating to people outside of it, but it doesn't have to be; if you like soda or ice cubes in your wine, be my guest.

SIPS NOT SHOTS

This should be your rule for spirits if you want to slow down the drinking and enjoy those units. We will look at how paying attention, smelling, and swirling slow down drinking wine; the same thing goes for spirits. Some whisky purists may say drink it neat, but others will say adding water releases more aromas. Whisky is diluted from cask strength with local water before it is bottled, as, at over 60 per cent alcohol, most people would struggle to appreciate the finer sides of the flavours. So don't feel you have to drink it straight up. Remember, we are drinking in a way that gives us the most pleasure.

EAT! WINE WITH FOOD, FOOD WITH WINE

Eat before you drink. Consuming food with wine slows down the rate at which it is absorbed, reducing your BAC compared to drinking on an empty stomach. The stomach is a lopsided pouch. When you drink with no food present, liquid slides down the flatter side of the stomach, straight through into the small intestine to be absorbed into the bloodstream. Drinking wine with a meal means the alcohol stays longer in the stomach; less alcohol reaches the small intestine, and some has time to be absorbed in the stomach. What does go into the small intestine does so at a slower rate, giving the liver time to work its magic.

Vinegar and cinnamon are thought to slow down gastric emptying, which might be behind the claims that cinnamon reduces blood sugar levels in diabetics and some of the health claims about cider vinegar. Drinking large volumes of liquid with meals, however, is not so good, as it accelerates gastric emptying. Fat is digested more slowly and slows gastric emptying time compared to carbohydrates—hence the sugar spike.

Blood alcohol levels are higher for people who drink sparkling wine with food, compared to the same amount of still wine. One theory is that the carbonation stimulates gastric emptying, reducing the time the alcohol remains in the stomach. Drinking with food also means you drink more slowly in between mouthfuls, increasing the pleasure, giving you time think about the wine a little more. Food and wine matching is fun, as the flavours of the food and the wine change with different pairings. Anything that calls for a little introspection and even discussion is going to slow down consumption.

Drinking on an empty stomach gets you drunk faster, and getting drunk faster can lead to more drinking as the night goes on. Eating something while you drink may help you make wiser food choices and should help avoid the drunken munchies. You know that irresistible starving feeling after a few drinks when you pass the pizza takeout on the way home. Eating after drinking is no help. Food has to be in your stomach before happy hour. Eating can also help prevent symptoms like nausea, upset stomach, and headaches.

SLEEP: NIX THE NIGHTCAP

Drinking may help you fall asleep faster, but it disrupts your sleep cycle, leading to sleep apnoea—obstructed breathing (and snoring). Breathing difficulties cause you to toss and turn, elevating stress hormones and making it harder to get back to sleep. You don't spend enough time in all-important REM (rapid eye movement) cycles, and you tend to wake up too soon. (REM cycles last between 90 and 110 minutes.[33]) If you've been drinking heavily, a hangover might strike in the last part of the night, leaving you too uncomfortable to get back to sleep.

Sleep is important; it's when the wear and tear gets repaired, physical and mental, as we produce the regenerative hormone melatonin and growth hormones. Sleeping less than eight hours a night can lead to weight gain; higher levels of ghrelin, a hormone that increases hunger; and lower levels of leptin, a hormone that suppresses hunger. In other words, using alcohol as a sleep aid only adds to a weight problem. Stop drinking (and eating) three or four hours before bedtime, and you'll lose weight more easily, sleep better, and have more energy (and willpower) the next day.

We mentioned the 4 a.m. hot and sweaty palpitations that women might put down to being of a certain age. Keep a note of what you drink and when and how you sleep, and you may be surprised. One bedtime tip that does help—drink water to fight dehydration.

THE HANGOVER

This probably merits a chapter all by itself, but I'm not going to give it the space, as the hangover is now going to be part of your past. The morning-after price of excess consumption can include a pounding headache, fatigue, dry mouth, a queasy stomach, and a weakened immune system; this is mainly caused by dehydration. As I mentioned earlier, alcohol is a diuretic, which is why small amounts can help the kidneys. Excess alcohol consumption soaks the water out of your system, causing you to urinate more. The queues in the ladies room at the bar are not just because we are reapplying lipstick!

This dehydration leaves you with a pounding headache. Drinking water and a good night's sleep are two of the cheapest beauty secrets. Match each glass of alcohol with at least one glass of water. This will also help with the morning-after dry mouth feeling exacerbated by the fact your saliva glands don't produce saliva during the night.

Tannins and other compounds, such as congeners found in whisky, can make a hangover worse. The gentlest choices are beer and clear spirits, such as vodka and gin. But they have a higher alcohol level than wine. Mixing spirits with fruit juice can be fattening (some juices such as pineapple have high sugar levels—ditch the pina coladas), but it may reduce the hangover.

A hangover, or the memory of one, is probably the greatest motivator for reasonable alcohol consumption, more and more so as the years fly by. That is the voice of experience talking!

Follow the advice above about late-night drinking and eating. Go to bed with a large glass of water and a liver-friendly tea. And you'll be smug in the morning. Worried about getting up in the night because you drank too much water before bed? Avoid evening diuretics such as green tea.

You can Google hangover cures, but the best cure is prevention. Having said that, here's a quick word of warning: Don't take acetaminophen (Tylenol) after a night of drinking; it's bad for the liver.

Coffee increases dehydration, and hair of the dog just postpones the pain and can lead to alcohol poisoning and a start on the slippery road to alcohol dependency. So, prevention it is then. There's nothing wrong with feeling fabulous and virtuous the next day.

MINDFULNESS

SAVOUR THE WINE, SAVOUR THE MOMENT

I'm a yogi. I love yoga (see chapter seven). One of the tenets of yoga is being present in the moment. So the idea of mindfulness, whether it's drinking, eating, or just being, is right up my street.

None of the reasons for reaching for a drink mentioned above are inherently wrong. What is important is to be aware of the choices you are making when you reach for a drink —this is mindfulness.

Is your motivation for drinking the pleasure of savouring a glass of lovely wine? Choosing a wine to complement a dish? Now you're talking.

Bearing that in mind, we want to make the most of those allocated units. We should choose carefully and not squander our valuable drinking resources. What about the practise? How are we going to put all this newfound knowledge to good use?

USE YOUR SENSES

Using our sense of smell and sense of sight when we are eating and drinking reduces our consumption. Our visual sense primes our senses of smell and taste. We process visual input ten times faster than we do olfactory. Out of sight is out of mind. Keep the bottles tucked away so they are not the first things you see when you walk in the kitchen. It's better for the wine, too, as wine should be kept in a cool dark place, preferably lying on its side if it has a cork. So you'll be doing the wine a favour as well as yourself. If you find yourself visualising the bottle or glass, open a book or turn the TV on.

SMELL THE WINE

When you decide to serve a glass of wine, take a look at it and smell it (more about tasting techniques later). Admiring the colour of the wine, swirling it around in the glass can tell us a lot about the wine we will be tasting. It heightens our anticipation of enjoyment, providing a little more delayed gratification. Our sense of smell is a valuable tool in moderation. Part of our satisfaction during eating and drinking comes from our sense of smell. Taste and smell are so closely linked; eating or drinking with a nose peg results in very little taste sensation or satisfaction. Taking time to smell the aromas of wine before and during drinking will increase the perception of satiety, and surprisingly enough, even if it smells delicious, you will drink less.

We'll work more on tasting skills so we can sniff and swirl our way to delayed gratification, moderation, and more intense drinking pleasure in chapter four.

I have talked (endlessly) about moderation. The key way to drink moderately without feeling like you are depriving yourself is to drink mindfully—drink with awareness. How?

We already mentioned the triggers that make us reach for a drink earlier in the chapter. Here are some steps to drinking mindfully:

- When you reach for a drink, ask yourself, why did I choose this? Is it what I really want now or is it what everyone else is drinking? Is this a habit or a decision?
- Smell the wine (chapter four). Enjoy the aromas. Delayed gratification and anticipation apply here, as well as mindfulness. Use your senses.
- Sip; don't gulp. Pick out those flavours and sensations. If you don't pay attention to aromas and tastes, you are missing out on the best bits of drinking.
- Then swallow. Put your glass down. Enjoy the sensation. It's like putting your knife and fork down between mouthfuls to give yourself the time to chew properly. (This is both good manners and good for the digestion; it allows your stomach to communicate satiety to the brain so you eat less). If you keep your glass in your hand, you will keep sipping, often for something to do.
- Do you really need another mouthful? Ask yourself, did I really enjoy that? Am I drinking because I'm thirsty or because I want to taste another mouthful of that lovely wine because it goes well with the food? Or is it because I'm nervous and don't know what to do with my hands?
- At the end of the glass, before automatically refilling, have a think about how much you enjoyed the experience and how it made you feel.

It's mindful drinking, but if you're in a social context don't get too carried away. It's supposed to be a social lubricant; you don't really want to be completely off on your own little cloud.

THE KISS PRINCIPLES FOR MODERATION

- I try and work to no more than two glasses of wine a day (can be replaced by a whisky, G&T or other cocktail as preferred).
- Take no fewer than two days off drinking per week.
- Drink (water) before you drink (alcohol).
- Eat before you drink.

MOTIVATION

- Take charge! Accept responsibility for your drinking habits—your life, your choices.
- Set yourself SMART goals.

AND MINDFULNESS

- Think before you drink.
- Be in the moment, savour, and enjoy.
- Make it last.

CHAPTER THREE

LOVE YOUR LIVER

WHY YOUR LIVER IS IMPORTANT AND WHY YOU SHOULD LOVE IT

UNDERSTANDING HOW OUR liver works will help us in deciding what changes we can make to help it to function as efficiently as possible. The French are obsessed with their livers, perhaps with due cause. The first time I heard the expression "mal au foie" (my liver hurts), I had no idea what the person was talking about. Feeling liverish or off colour (green?) is probably the English equivalent. Or perhaps the best equivalent is the typical English understatement "feeling a bit under the weather" (hung-over). The liver is not the only part of the body that works to eliminate alcohol, but it processes about 80 per cent of the alcohol we consume.

Alcohol, along with food, passes from the stomach into the small intestine and, from there, into the bloodstream and on to the liver, all within about five minutes. Once there, it is broken down by the enzyme alcohol dehydrogenase into water and carbon dioxide. It takes about an hour to break down the alcohol from a single drink.

Too much alcohol, and the enzyme can't keep up with its detox function; the excess alcohol is changed into acetaldehyde, an acidic and toxic chemical, causing symptoms we associate with a hangover—headache, nausea, tiredness, sore muscles, and so on.

Not everyone processes alcohol at the same speed. Our genes define the concentration and type of enzymes in our livers; they vary in different populations. This concentration affects the rate of alcohol breakdown, the reaction to alcohol, and the resulting by-products. It explains why certain people flush, while others get tipsy quickly and some are more or less susceptible to alcoholism and liver disease.

We can't change our genes, but we can look at other things that affect our ability to process alcohol. How quickly alcohol is absorbed into the blood, distributed, metabolised, and excreted is affected by different factors, including:

- Drinking patterns—how much and how quickly you drink
- The type of alcoholic beverage
- Diet and the presence of food in the stomach
- Age
- Smoking
- Environmental factors
- Gender
- Even the time of day

A way of keeping the liver and the digestion efficient is not to overload it with too much work. Moderate alcohol consumption of course, but this isn't the only thing you can do to protect your liver. Our digestive system takes what we swallow, absorbs nutrients, protects us from poison, and excretes the leftovers that are of no value. The liver plays the leading role in this complex system and should be treated with a bit of respect if we want it to function well. As well as alcohol, the liver detoxifies other harmful substances that enter the body through air, water, food, or skin.

Situated to the right of the stomach, the liver is the body's largest detox gland. It's a busy organ, helping to control sugar levels; purifying the blood from other toxins, drugs, and hormones; and storing some vitamins and iron. Reducing your intake of all toxins will reduce the burden on the liver.

Your liver also produces bile, which helps dissolve fat. Drinking a lot of alcohol with a fatty meal slows that process down, too. It's useful to know what other substances, aside from alcohol, put stress on the liver.

THINGS THAT INCREASE THE LIVER'S WORKLOAD

Sugar. Too much sugar isn't only going to make you fat. It contributes to inflammation, rots your teeth, and can harm your liver. The liver converts sugar into fat. Too much refined sugar and high-fructose corn syrup causes a fatty build-up that can lead to liver disease. You are going to have to choose your "poison". Sugar addiction can be as difficult to get through as alcoholism.

Drugs. The liver processes most medications, so the same rule of overloading applies, as the liver enzyme responsible for alcohol metabolism also works on many medications. Drinking can make certain drugs less effective, as the liver will not process them optimally. This is one reason many medications come with the warning not to drink while you are taking them. Propranolol (which is prescribed for the treatment of hypertension and disturbances of the heart rhythm), the pain medication acetaminophen, the blood thinner warfarin, and the sedative diazepam are a few examples. Even common pain relievers should be taken with care, as overdosing on anything that has acetaminophen can harm your liver. Some drugs are particularly dangerous bedfellows of alcohol. For example, mixing alcohol and acetaminophen or paracetamol can cause acute liver failure, and alcohol and aspirin taken together increase the risk of gastric bleeding. Alcohol increases analgesic effects, reinforcing the sedative effects of opiates.

If you're taking any medication, make sure you talk to your doctor or pharmacist about any reactions that may result from mixing it with alcohol. And always pay close attention to contraindications on the packet or instructions.

Additives. Some additives in our foods are considered poisons by the body. MSG (monosodium glutamate) for example has been linked with obesity and inflammation within the body, particularly the liver.[34] Choosing fresh, organic, unprocessed food as much as much as possible will reduce strain on the liver from additives. The jury is out as to how damaging some of these chemicals are in terms of the development of cancer and other degenerative diseases. My theory is this: If in doubt, don't wherever possible.

Trans fats. Trans fats are man-made fats present in many packaged foods and baked goods, often listed as "partially hydrogenated". They make your liver work extra hard to process them, cause inflammation, and make you fat—none of which is good news.

Smoking. I don't think this needs much of an explanation. Tobacco smoke contains toxins, which means more work for the liver. Don't do it. If you enjoy a cigarette with your drink, be aware that smoking and drinking together increases the risk of oesophageal and laryngeal cancer by activating many pro-carcinogens found in tobacco smoke. We know that self-control is more difficult after a drink or two, so if you are trying to give up cigarettes, you might want to stay away from the drink for a while. Tobacco use also may increase the risk of osteoporosis and fractures, with the combination of smoke and alcohol compounding osteoporosis risk. So again that ciggie with your drink is a definite no.

It's a social thing. If everyone around you is having a cigarette with his or her wine, you'll be more tempted. Remove the trigger.

Excess vitamin A. Vitamin A is really important for health, but you can have too much of a good thing. Vitamin A helps improve vision, strengthens bones, and gives a boost to your immune system. It is found naturally in eggs and milk, as well as in plants such as fresh fruits and vegetables, especially those that are red, orange, and yellow. I'm a big fan of supplements (see below), but please check the levels of Vitamin A you are consuming. Recommended doses of vitamin A are around 150 mg or about 10,000 IU per day. More than this can be harmful for your liver. The same enzymes that break down alcohol break down excess vitamin A. Check with your doctor before you take any extra vitamin A. Moderation in all things.

WHEN DOES THE LIVER WORK?

Remember that with all this metabolic activity, the liver is the hottest organ in the body. It's at its busiest at about 4 a.m. This explains why, after an evening of overindulgence, night sweats and that groggy half-awake feeling often happen around this time. You may think that a little nightcap before bed is just the thing to help you sleep, and it might well help you nod off. But drinking before bed could be what is waking you up before dawn.

LIVER DISEASE

It's common knowledge that excess alcohol consumption causes liver damage. In processing and breaking down alcohol, the liver can become first fatty and then hard. This is known as alcohol-induced fatty liver disease

(ALD). You might like the French delicacy of foie gras with your glass of Sauternes, but you really don't want one inside your system.

Alcohol is not the only cause of liver disease. A diet high in sugar and fat can lead to non-alcoholic fatty liver disease (NAFLD). The swollen liver can harden and create scar tissue (cirrhosis). You are more susceptible to NAFLD if you are overweight, middle-aged, or have diabetes.

The liver needs lots of oxygen to break down alcohol. With excess alcohol to be processed, certain areas can be deprived of oxygen, causing liver damage through oxidative stress, which can lead to DNA damage and may, thereby, play an important role in alcohol-related development of liver cancer.[35]

In the Greek myth of Prometheus, the power of his liver to regenerate every night after being devoured every day by an eagle is put down to Prometheus's godlike immortality, but our livers do have their own bit of immortality. The liver is the only visceral organ that can regenerate, replacing damaged tissue with new cells within about thirty days.

Why does the liver have this unique talent? As the main site of detoxification in the body, it is exposed to many toxins, which can cause cell death in the process. This regeneration capacity is not an excuse to treat the liver with disrespect; continued attacks on the liver will prevent complete regeneration, creating scar tissue and cirrhosis, and it will eventually become too scarred to function properly. If you stop drinking alcohol early enough, lose some weight, and start exercising, some liver damage may be reversible—healing can begin as early as a few days to weeks after ceasing alcohol use. If the damage is too severe, healing may take months and may not be reversible at all.

HOW HEALTHY IS YOUR LIVER?

If your answers to the tests in the last chapter were worrying, you should consider taking a closer look at your liver. The most common symptoms of liver failure are very non-specific. They include fatigue, achy muscles, itchy skin, excessive tiredness, and lack of drive that you might be putting down to something else. More worrying signs are jaundice or yellowing of the eyes and skin, dark urine, very pale or light coloured stools, swelling in your belly, bleeding from the gut, mental confusion, and retention of fluids in the abdomen.

Hepatitis, normally associated with viral infections, is a generic term for inflammation and damage to liver cells, caused by drugs, toxins, alcohol, inherited diseases, certain metabolic diseases, and viruses. These viruses are called A, B, C, D, E, and G; the most common causes are hepatitis A, B, and C. They are not lifestyle related, except for some that can be sexually transmitted, but that is beyond the realms of this book. If you feel you have an issue with your liver, get a check-up from your doctor. A simple blood test can measure levels of liver enzymes in your blood; you can also undertake a gamma GT (liver function) test or a fibro scan. This will allow you to spot any possible damage. As we have seen, if damage is spotted early enough, lifestyle changes can dramatically affect your chances of recovery. Don't wait.

THE LIVER'S LITTLE HELPERS

I love French pharmacies; they are a treasure trove of traditional cures, as well as all the wonderful cosmetics, lotions, and potions. You can find herbal teas and tinctures for everything from "heavy legs" to clear skin to liver tonics. We've looked at toxins to avoid. Now here are a few things that can help liver function.

A bitter pill. Many liver cures taste bitter, and for good reason. Bitterness signals poison, which puts the liver on full alert to process and eliminate them. Bitter elements in a diet have long been considered a liver tonic, stimulating and encouraging the liver to kick in and work harder and even regenerating hepatocytes (liver cells).

The Eeyore principle. Milk thistle (Chardon-Marie) is one of the few substances thought to stimulate hepatocyte regeneration. Artichokes, another member of the thistle family, are also a traditional liver tonic, especially in Bordeaux where the "artichauts de Macau" are a famous speciality of the Medoc. Perhaps it's no coincidence they are grown in one of the top wine areas of the region?

Liver teas and tonics. Dandelion, burdock, wormwood, dried Berberis (barberry) bark, and yarrow all encourage the function of the liver if you can find them—and get past their … acquired taste. Can anyone else remember drinking dandelion and burdock as a child? Just like root beer and sarsaparilla, it is now known as a soda, but their origins are as liver tonics. Have a chat to your local pharmacist about liver tonics. I'm sure they'll have some bitter drops for you to place on your tongue before meals.

Supplementary help: Multivitamins. I know this is a little controversial but I'm a big believer in taking a good multivitamin. Despite valiant efforts, I rarely eat as healthy and as balanced a diet as I should (more on this matter in chapter six). Depending on what you read, you should consume six to ten portions of fruit and veg a day. But do you really? I don't. Well not always. I'm full of good intentions; breakfast is usually exemplary, but it's often downhill from there, especially when I'm travelling. I'm also sceptical about the quality of a lot of food we eat, the state of our soils, and the length of the food chain. In his book *Diet for a New America*, John Robbins explains how soil depletion of trace elements causes a lack of certain essential minerals in our diet.[36] He does say cocoa is grown in tropical locations that are still nutrient rich—just saying! Consequently, I take multivitamins to compensate. Oh, and dark chocolate.

Drinking alcohol depletes or hampers the absorption of some essential nutrients, so supplementation for people who drink is even more important. It helps compensate for the lack of absorption, in addition to supporting the liver. It doesn't get you off the hook from healthy eating and is not an excuse to skimp on your fruit and veg. Eating regular and large portions of fruit and veg is the surest and safest way to ensure that you can combat some of the negative side effects of drinking, as well as being generally good for your health. Getting the majority of our vitamins and minerals from real food ensures a better absorption due to interactions in their natural forms that just may not work in supplement form. Scientists still don't completely understand how it works.

Having said that, I see taking good quality supplements as an insurance policy, and they seem to suit me. If you have any doubts as to whether you need or should be taking supplements, get a blood test to see what vitamins you may or may not be lacking. Vitamin D (the sunshine vitamin), for example, is often on the most-needed list, as are B vitamins. (Marmite anyone?) Vitamin C is a key vitamin in protection against illness and infection, and it may help to prevent cancer, too. It is abundant in most fresh fruit and veg, but less than two portions a day and you are not getting your daily quota.

Antioxidants. It's not just vitamins and minerals we may need to supplement. Other elements that may be missing from our diet are antioxidants, polyphenols produced by plants that help combat signs of ageing by mopping up free radicals in our body. Free radicals are unstable molecules produced as a by-product of chemical reactions in the body. Missing an electron, they can cause oxidative stress, leading to inflammation and disease if not held in check by antioxidants. Happily, as well as in fruit and veg, these seem to be abundant in red wine. More to follow.

The supplements I take are from the range of Lifeplus[37], recommended to me by a friend who is a doctor as well as a winemaker. Their wine-based backstory resonates with me. Lifeplus's leading product is an antioxidant complex called Proanthanols. Based on OPCs, (oligomeric proanthocyanidins, since you ask) extracted from grape seeds and certain types of pine bark found in Southern France. Dr Masquelier discovered them at the University of Bordeaux in the 1940s. (You can see why I liked the story.) OPCs are naturally occurring antioxidant substances found in plants known as polyphenolic flavonoids. They are present in hundreds of plants, but grape seeds and pine bark seem to be particularly good sources. Handy that, as we have lots of both in the South West of France.

Tree bark might not sound very tasty, but it's nothing new. In the winter of 1534 to 1535, after months at sea without fresh fruit and veg, French explorer Jacques Cartier's ship's crew was dying of scurvy. Upon arriving in the new world, on advice from locals, he gave his dying crew tea made from the needles and bark of pine trees. Incredibly, the men recovered completely within a week.

Glutathione is a key antioxidant that helps the liver process alcohol-induced toxins like acetaldehyde. I first heard about glutathione in winemaking; it is an antioxidant found naturally in grapes and is especially important in the making of white wine. Unlike red wine, white wines do not contain high levels of tannins and other polyphenols leached from the skins of grapes during fermentation. These tannins are antioxidants (see polyphenols above) protecting red wine from oxidation. Many white wines are particularly sensitive to oxidation, their aromatic complexity and freshness being their signature. Winemakers carefully monitor and optimise levels of glutathione by picking early, before overripeness occurs, and ensuring nitrogen levels in the soil.

Good news: This means white wines have health benefits just as red wines do! You can also take glutathione as a supplement if you think you might have a heavy night ahead. The jury is out as to whether consuming it directly works. [38] Eggs contain cysteine, which can also be broken down by the body into glutathione. This may explain why a cooked breakfast is considered a hangover cure.

The alpha and omega. An excess of fat in the diet can put strain on the liver, which needs to produce bile to break fat down into a digestible form.

We need some fat for our health, and just as with alcohol, not all fats are created equal. The fats we really need to function well are omega fats. There are two types—6 and 3. Omega-6 fats are just about everywhere, especially in processed oils such as rapeseed (canola) and sunflower seed oil. The trickier fats to find are the 3s. The ideal ratio of omega-6 to omega-3 is considered to be somewhere between 2:1 and 1:1. It would seem we are all overdosing on the 6s at the expense of 3s. Fish oil is a good source but has a similar effect to that of aspirin, so if you are on anticoagulants, supplementing with it may prolong bleeding time. Consult your doctor before you begin taking it if you have any doubts at all. Fish oils often contain Vitamin A, and as we saw earlier, high doses of vitamin A are toxic to the liver. If you are unsure of what levels are in supplements you are taking, or if you are taking several different supplements, check with your doctor to make sure you are not exceeding the recommended levels of 10,000 IU or 150 mg a day.

Read more about what fats to concentrate on in chapter six.

Folate, a B vitamin, is very important for growth, especially cell division and building DNA, which is why it is recommended for pregnant women. Current thinking is that folate may help prevent cancer by preventing errors in DNA replication. As alcohol blocks the absorption of folate and inactivates it in the blood and tissues, all drinkers should ensure their diets are rich in fruits and vegetables to get enough folate and other B vitamins. The link to folate absorption could be one of the clues to breast cancer being linked to alcohol consumption—research is still being carried out. Folate may also help reduce the risk of colon cancer in alcohol drinkers. Good sources include green vegetables (especially asparagus, broccoli, Brussels sprouts, spinach, and spring greens, cauliflower), soy flour, many varieties of beans, and liver.

Pro and prebiotics. The whole digestive system plays a role in detoxing. A healthy digestive tract eliminates toxins efficiently, taking some of the pressure off the liver. Have you ever had an upset tummy after a heavy night? Alcohol can be just as much of an enemy to our gut flora as stress or even antibiotics, leading to disruptions in our gut microbiome and increased intestinal permeability (leaky gut). [39] Alcohol can also multiply the number of gas-producing bacteria by a factor of up to 1,000. You have been warned!

Our microbiomes deserve to be treated with as much tender loving care as our livers. Not only does the gut microbiome help digest the food we eat, reduce bloating and neutralising toxins, but it also produces vitamins, and even helps raise our mood. More about how to help this population in chapter six.

Coffee. Surprisingly, drinking coffee (no more than four cups per day) has been linked to lower levels of liver cirrhosis in both drinkers and non-drinkers, indicating that coffee may have some protective properties—those polyphenols again. Not everything we love is bad for us.

Ginger. Known as a soothing or carminative (gas relieving) food, ginger helps speed up the digestive process and is good for easing nausea. You can drink it as a tea or use it fresh in a stir-fry.

Peppermint. Peppermint leaf and oil also help relax stomach muscles and relieve digestive complaints. A cup of peppermint tea after dinner works wonders.

THE KISS PRINCIPLES TO MAKE YOUR LIVER FEEL LOVED

- If you are drinking, don't overload the body with other toxins for the liver to cope with: Avoid sugar, excess fats, medications, etc.
- Take a good multimineral/multivitamin complex/antioxidant.
- Top up your gut flora with prebiotics and probiotics.
- Include omega-3s in your diet or take them as oils or supplements.
- If you are planning a night where you risk going over your two-glass limit, take glutathione or milk thistle before and after to give your liver a helping hand.

CHAPTER FOUR
HOW TO DRINK LIKE A FRENCH WOMAN

T HERE ARE SO many books about the wonderful French lifestyle—
telling us how all French women are slim and beautiful, with perfect
chic style; look ten years younger than their age; have perfect children
and great sex lives; and on and on and on. You name it, the French are better
at it than us. It's enough to make you reach for a drink!

I've lived in France for over thirty years. Let me dispel just a few myths
so that we non-French women can dust off our self-esteem. For a start, the
French have some great phrases relating to the after-effects of over indulgence,
such as "mal aux cheveux" (my hair hurts) and the famous "crise de foie" (a
liver crisis). So they obviously don't have this thing covered, either. If you
want to see French women of all shapes and sizes, just call in to my local
supermarket on a Saturday morning. All your insecurities will be put to rest.
Then again, European statistics do tell us that British women are the fourth
fattest of Europe—over 50 per cent are deemed overweight or obese—whereas
the French come in at number twenty-three with just over 40 per cent.[40]
Overweight Americans represent two out of three adults.[41]

When I first moved to Paris in the '80s, the "food revolution" hadn't hit
the United Kingdom. France didn't need a food revolution; the French were
passionate about good food, not in a trendy foodie way but in an "it's part
of my life" way. Good, fresh, seasonal, and varied food, prepared daily and

served to the family around the table was just what you did. And they still do it, often twice a day.

I was lucky enough to be brought up this way, too. My mother was a fabulous cook from a farming background. My grandfather was a farmer and the village butcher and publican, and my grandmother was a poultry farmer. Fresh home-prepared food was something I took for granted.

When I was writing my CV on leaving university in the United Kingdom, my tutor told me not to include a love of food in my list of interests—too "lotus eating". Well it didn't worry the French; I was now in the land of the lotus eaters. The variety of food available in France, and of course the accompanying wines, made my inner foodie feel right at home. Back in England, my contemporaries were putting deposits down on their first flats. In Paris, everyone rented their homes, spending their money on the food on the table and the clothes on their backs. Unsurprisingly, I was getting larger and larger; my expanding waistline and student budget would not allow for the clothes. But the food, well, no problem. It's not just French women who get fat when they leave France; it works the other way around, too!

In my thirty years in the French food and booze business, I've had time to look at the French relationship with alcohol. Based on experience, not sound market research, I was convinced that the French drank less and in a more civilised way than the Brits. I've organised many events for a mixed British/French crowd over the years, and French caterers would always increase their allowance of alcohol when I told them Brits were involved, expecting per head consumption to outstrip their normal calculations.

WHO IS DRINKING WHAT?

We know everybody lies about his or her alcohol consumption, but figures from the World Health Organization (WHO) show that the French, in fact, don't drink less than the rest of us. These figures date a bit (they're from 2010), and may have a bias, as they are from a report concerning substance abuse, but they make for interesting reading.[42] Expressed in equivalent litres of pure alcohol consumed across all categories, France wins at 12.2 litres per capita, with the United Kingdom at 11.6 and the United States at 9.2. What is interesting is what we drink. In France, 56.4 per cent of that alcohol is consumed as wine, compared to 33.8 per cent in the UK and only 17.3 per cent in the US.

So, yes the French drink. But it's mainly wine, which is hardly surprising when they make so much. The WHO figures estimate a margin for under-reporting (lying) about how much reporters drink, but they also show the divide between men and women. In the United States, men are reported as drinking 13.6 litres per capita per year and women 4.9. In the United Kingdom, it's 16.5 litres for men and 6.9 for women. The French beat us all at 17.8 litres for each man and 7.1 per woman.

That puts paid to my theory that French woman don't drink as much as English women. But they are very good at putting on a sober front, and I'm not the only one who thinks so. Twice, driving home in rural France, the gendarmes have pulled us over to be breathalysed. Fortunately, neither time my husband was over the limit. But he must have been close, as each time the gendarme kindly suggested that perhaps Madame should drive home. He didn't breathalyse me. Those clever French women definitely have a sober image. I've attended many a French dinner party where the women just dip their lips into the wine without really imbibing. Perhaps French men make sure their partners are the designated drivers, or perhaps they are all closet drinkers. More research needs to be done!

The French may not drink less, but they do drink differently; they consume the majority of their alcohol as wine and mainly at meal times. Friends rarely meet for drink in France. They're not antisocial; they drink with food, so they'll meet you for dinner or lunch. Yes they are the champions of the "aperitif" but very much as a pre-meal experience—no preloading here.

BINGE-DRINKING

This is another area where the British feel we are champions. Binge-drinking is not falling down drunk in the streets. Officially, binge-drinking is considered as five or more drinks for men and four or more drinks for women in about two hours. The WHO report politely refers to this as "heavy episodic drinking" and claims that 16.2 per cent of the US population binge-drink (24.7 per cent of men and 7.5 per cent of women), as do 29.8 per cent of the French (45 per cent of men and 14.4% per cent of women). That's more than the Brits at 27 per cent, but this figure includes 37.2 per cent of men and 16.8 per cent of women.[43] This is where British women live up to our reputation as party animals then.

So with a Gaelic shrug, we Brits can finally shake off that image of being the alcoholics of Europe and sip our wine over dinner with our continental cousins. Most of my French girlfriends, even those who don't work in the business, wouldn't dream of having a lunch or dinner with friends without a glass of wine. Mind you that describes most of my girlfriends, wherever they come from, so perhaps that's more to do with my choice of friends rather than national drinking habits. Moving swiftly along.

The secret is wine with food and food with wine, regular and moderate (see chapter two). The traditional way of drinking wine in most wine-producing areas is with food. The lovely complexity of wine is enhanced by food, and food is enhanced by wine. We have already seen how drinking with food is better for us, as the combination slows down the absorption of alcohol into the bloodstream. Food and wine matching is a passionate subject. Many books[44] have been written about it. The subject is much too interesting to get into in enough detail here, but to sum up—the lighter the food, the lighter the wine and vice versa. But if you like a big bold red with fish, who am I to say don't do it? Again, your wine, your choice.

Moderate wine drinkers tend to have lower mortality rates and healthier hearts, [45] but moderate drinking with meals delivers maximum health benefits. Wine and eating go better together![46]

FRENCH WOMEN AND EATING HABITS

French women drink wine with food, but their eating habits are worth a look, too:

- French women do not snack in between meals.
- Croissants are for breakfast, not for a mid-morning top up.
- You don't see French women walking around town with polystyrene cups of milky coffee. In fact, apart from breakfast, they never put milk in coffee.
- They eat three meals a day.
- They don't eat on the hoof; they stop for lunch, take their time, eat slowly, and enjoy.
- They don't eat half a baguette while waiting for the starter to arrive or a bowl of peanuts with the aperitif.
- They drink lots of water.

- They eat their veg; a French family meal will usually start with either salad (crudités) in the summer or soup in the winter. Vegetables are served with the main course and salad offered with cheese before dessert.
- They finish their meal with a strong (bitter) espresso, which closes the appetite.

In France, the advice before heading somewhere where there will be drink but no food is to take a spoonful of olive oil. In England, we advise a glass of milk. I prefer full-fat yoghurt, as it helps with those probiotics, too.

Take your time over meals, chewing well. You will eat less and enjoy it more. Chewing warns the stomach what food is heading its way, preparing the digestive process and allowing time for a full sensation to reach the brain from the stomach. This process slows down both food and wine consumption.

Start with water and continue. Drink at least one glass of water for every glass of wine. Headaches associated with hangovers are exacerbated by the dehydration as your body tries to dilute the alcohol. Help it!

WHAT IS GOOD WINE?

That is a very good question. A good wine is a wine you enjoy; understanding what you enjoy is the key. There are many great wine courses you can go on if you want to learn more. I highly recommend the WSET (Wine and Spirits Education Trust) courses as a good place to start. WSET has teachers all over the world; you can find one near you on the organisation's website.[47] In the meantime, here's a 101 of wine tasting to get you started on paying attention to what is in your wine glass.

A WORD ABOUT WINE TASTING

Paying attention to what we are drinking and taking the time to appreciate what is in the glass increases satisfaction and drinking pleasure and slows consumption—all things we are trying to accomplish.

If we choose our wine well, we can be confident that someone has gone to a lot of trouble and effort to produce that wine for us. So paying a little attention to what we're drinking seems only polite. It's not about wine snobbery but, rather, about understanding what is in the glass and, more importantly, whether you like it or not. Understanding what you like prevents disappointment and possibly expensive mistakes. You decide what you like. Don't let anyone else tell you what wine you should and shouldn't like (that goes for so many things in life). But don't be afraid to experiment and try new wines. You might discover a whole new passion.

For a brief introduction to wine tasting, please see the annex at the end of the book.

Please don't become a wine snob; there's nothing more boring. And there's no right or wrong in wine, unless a particular wine has a major fault. Just because it's more expensive doesn't always means it's better. But please avoid really cheap wine; once you've counted the price of a bottle, a label, the cork or screw cap (we love screw caps), taxes, transport, and retail margins, you need to be paying enough to ensure that there's money left for the content. Drink less, drink better.

If you need any more motivation, learning to taste may be good for the brain.[48] It has been likened to a sensory gym. Scientists compared master sommeliers' brains to those of a control group and found that the sommeliers had a "thicker" sensory area and a thicker memory area—and the areas were most active during tasting. Training your palate to taste might just be enhancing the brain as well as increasing your pleasure and may even help prevent neurodegenerative diseases. Exercise that grey matter by tasting. It's more fun than the crossword!

THE KISS PRINCIPLES TO DRINK LIKE A FRENCH WOMAN

- Don't snack between meals.
- Drink good wine, with good food.
- Take your time.
- Drink your coffee black.

CHAPTER FIVE
A DAILY DETOX

THERE IS A trend for dry January or February (it's a shorter month after all), giving your liver a rest by abstaining from alcohol for a month. It might give you a virtuous glow but perhaps, more importantly, it proves that you can control your alcohol consumption rather than the other way around. Beware: Taking a month off might make you feel less guilty, but it should not be an excuse to plunge back in to overdrinking with a clear conscience.

I'm not a fan of dry January (unless it's the odd dry martini), but I am all for having a few days a week off from drinking alcohol, just to prove to myself that I can. You would be surprised at how many people baulk at the thought of a day without a drink. Ouch, is that a bit close to home? I sympathise. When I went on my very first detox retreat, about twenty years ago, I couldn't remember the last time I had been a single day without a drink. I found it surprisingly easy, mainly as I was away from my usual triggers (see above). I found the chocolate deprivation harder to endure, but it did give me time to reassess how much I drank on a regular basis.

Detoxing is fashionable, but the body does a pretty good job of detoxing all by itself if you let it and even give it a helping hand. Without turning into a monk and licking water off the side of a cave, there are things we can do every day to help our body's natural detox function. Aside from not drinking too much, here are a few detox tools you might want to incorporate into your daily routine.

A MORNING DETOX ROUTINE

Drink! Drink a glass of water at room temperature even before you get out of bed. I leave a large glass of water on my bedside table when I go to bed. Then, as soon as I wake, I sit up and drink it.

Stretch. You know those cartoons when people wake up and stretch. How many people really do that? If you don't, you should. Sit on the side of the bed and reach your hands up to the celling and clasp your hands. Stretch over to the right and left and then try to bring them down behind your head and neck and pull up and out of the waist and open the heart up to the ceiling. Feels good, right?

Oil pulling. Oil pulling is a traditional Ayurveda practise, which claims to increase oral hygiene, reduce gum inflammation, and keep teeth white. Take a small teaspoon of coconut or sesame oil in your mouth. The temperature of your mouth will make the coconut oil melt. Swish it around for about two minutes or so. It's called pulling, as you pull the oil backwards and forwards through the mouth. If you can't bear the taste, add a few drops of peppermint into the bottle.

Why? Overnight, your saliva production slows. Swishing oil around the mouth encourages saliva production, which has a cleansing effect, important for preventing infection around teeth and gums but also for keeping bad bacteria from proliferating. Coconut oil is rich in lauric acid, a fatty acid with antibacterial, antimicrobial, and antifungal properties. Emulsified with saliva, it gets in between teeth and reaches part of the mouth that regular brushing doesn't. Some research shows that bacterial infection from the mouth can have a harmful effect on the heart. Peppermint is also good for your digestion, so it's a win-win. Stained teeth are another side effect of wine tasting, so this practice is a lifesaver for me.

Does that sound too time consuming in the morning? I usually multitask (it's a girl thing), swishing away while I'm body brushing.

Body brushing. The liver might be the major detox organ of the body, but the skin also detoxes, mainly through sweat, eliminating toxins along with water. Body brushing stimulates the circulation of the lymph just under skin. Your lymph is a parallel circulatory system to blood, moving mainly fats and some waste products from metabolism. Unlike blood, it doesn't have the heart at its centre but relies on your movement and muscle activity to work—another reason to keep moving and exercise (more on that later).

Body brushing helps stimulate this system and gets it started first thing in the morning.

How do you body brush? You can find body brushes for sale, but a soft brush, shower mitt or loofah will do. Use light movements from the extremities, and brush towards the heart. Move from the feet up the legs and from the hands up the arms on the torso towards the heart. Then go over the stomach and gut in a clockwise circular movement, just to give your digestive system a little boost too. I do this first thing in the morning before a shower. It really wakes you up and gives your skin a glow. It exfoliates the skin too—another multitasker and a great start to the day.

Kick-start your digestion. Lemon juice dissolved in hot water first thing in the morning stimulates digestion and the liver and kick-starts the system. Add a slice of fresh ginger, a pinch of turmeric, and a screw of pepper (pepper and turmeric are absorbed better when consumed together), and you have three major antioxidants that also offer protection against colds and infections. Try to drink this within a half hour of waking and a half hour before eating breakfast.

If this sound like too much to do first thing in the morning, you can prep it the night before; put the lemon, ginger, and spices in the bottom of a mug with just enough hot water to cover, leave it with a saucer on top, and then just add boiling water in the morning. It will taste even better, as the ginger will have had time to infuse. You'll be addicted in no time. When I'm in our home in Mauritius, I can easily find fresh turmeric root. But beware; turmeric stains your fingers so you look like a chain smoker. Powdered, as long as it hasn't been hanging around too long, will do just fine. Some of my friends also add apple cider vinegar or have a blend of apple cider vinegar and honey at the start of the day. I prefer using it in salad dressing, but give it a try to see if it suits you. Some claim apple cider vinegar is good for achy joints, but that joint pain can also be a result of dehydration if you have been drinking the night before.

AND AN EVENING ROUTINE

The liver is a remarkable organ; it can regenerate itself. But to do so, it needs a rest now and again. Although I'm not a big fan of intensive detoxes or fasts, as I mentioned above, I am a believer in a daily detox or fast. Experiments since the 1930s have shown that the lifespan of rats and worms can be extended through calorie restriction.[49] The jury is out as to whether this works for humans. During fasting, fat storage stops in favour of fat burning and repair. While the body is not busy digesting, which consumes a lot of energy and produces a lot of toxins, it can get on with other jobs, including eliminating those toxins and repair. Rejuvenation starts taking place, but prolonged fasting can also lead to muscle loss, which, in the long term, reduces metabolic rate. This means, as soon as you start eating again, even sensibly, you put on weight. The solution? Intermittent fasting, the theory behind the famous 5:2 diet.[50]

A night fast. What I am proposing is basically night fasting. Try and give your body a break of at least ten, and if possible twelve, hours between your last meal at night and breakfast the next morning. Basically, that means don't eat late at night, and stop eating at least three hours before going to sleep.

A night fast will:

- Detox your body (autophagy)
- Keep weight under control, since the later you eat, the less chance you have of burning up some of the calories you have consumed before they are stored as fat
- Help you sleep better, and sleep detoxes the brain – On a full stomach, your sleep will be disturbed, and your system will be sluggish.
- Give your system a break from digesting, which is exhausting for the body, producing lots of free radicals
- Enable your body to concentrate on repairing itself and other activities

Eating early may not sound very sociable, especially in France where getting people over to dinner before 8.30 p.m. is almost impossible. If hanging out with friends for dinner is how you see people, this may sound unworkable, but give it some headspace. You don't have to do it every single night. Just try it when you can. When you're at home, eat earlier and lighter in the evening and see how much better you feel.

If you can't eat early, eat light. The rule I try and work by is no white food, in other words, no carbs (rice, pasta, potatoes, bread, and such) in the evening. It's usually what we reach for when we've been drinking, persuading ourselves that it'll soak up the booze and slowing down the absorption of alcohol, all helped by diminished self-control after a few drinks. You now know it's too late; if you want to slow down the absorption of alcohol, you have to eat before drinking, not afterwards.

I don't find eating light in the evening a hardship. I'm a lady who lunches. My work and social life involve lots of lunches. If I've had a decent lunch, I really don't need a big dinner. Try it and see if your sleep improves, as well as your waistline.

Sleep it off. I believe the three best beauty secrets are a good night's sleep, lots of water, and a smile, none of which is expensive to implement. We'll talk about water later; if you get a good night's sleep, the smile should come a lot easier. Insomnia is an issue for many people, and eating early and light should help. A nightcap may help you to nod off, but it might not help you sleep through the night, especially if it adds another couple of units after a heavy evening. Remember your liver usually kicks in at about 4 a.m. (see chapter four). If you are starving, stave off the hunger pangs with a liver-friendly herbal tea.

Sleeping better reduces weight gain. Studies by David F. Dinges, PhD, professor of psychology at the Perelman School of Medicine in Pennsylvania showed that sleep deprivation not only makes you hungrier but also slows down your metabolic rate. [51]

On the subject of sleep, if you can sleep on your back, please do. It's one of the best wrinkle prevention techniques ever. Sleeping on your side scrunches up your face and upper chest and reinforces those lines. Sleeping on a silk pillow is supposed to help, but I haven't tried it—yet.

Part of your evening detox routine can be to wrap a hot water bottle in a towel and place it on your liver when to go to bed. The liver is on the right hand side of your body just by the bottom of the rib cage. The theory is this increases blood flow through the liver and heats it up, giving it an extra boost to action. This is a traditional remedy. You can also try a castor oil pack, but that's a little messier.

No raw after four. Another simple rule that was rammed into me at the Mayr Clinic[52] was "no raw after four." The digestive system slows down at night when we sleep. In the evening, you're not the only one who feels weary; your digestive system does too. It's a lot less effective later in the day. Raw veg is really difficult to digest and puts an enormous amount of strain on the system, so give it a break by eating cooked food in the evening. This is a tough one for me; my go-to meal, especially when I'm busy or feeling lazy, is to throw together a salad. To make it easy, I make a big batch of vegetable soup when I have time. I use a slow cooker to make stock once a week and then add in veg and freeze it in portions, so I can defrost as and when I need it. It's even easier than making salad and helps with hydration.

WATER THERAPY

Drinking enough water is an important part of detoxing, as it helps flush any toxins out of the body. We all know that we should be drinking regular amounts of water. Don't we? We are mainly water after all—on average 60 per cent by weight for an adult male and 55 per cent for an adult female. Remember one of the theories why women can drink less alcohol is the fact they have less body water to dilute it. Water makes up about 83 per cent of blood, 73 per cent of muscles, 25 per cent of body fat, and 22 per cent of bones. It is the medium in which most of the metabolic functions of the body take place and how enzymes move around and blood flows. Water regulates body temperature and lubricates joints. Severe dehydration can affect digestion, cause constipation, and dry out the skin, accentuating wrinkles.

An upside to drinking water is that it helps with weight loss; studies show that, by drinking water, people tended to eat and drink fewer calories, probably because the water filled them up. As a result, they lost weight. Often what we think of as hunger pangs is really thirst.

However, fizzy water is not so helpful. The carbon dioxide may increase the level of the hunger hormone ghrelin, causing us to eat more. So ask, "Am I hungry, or am I thirsty?" Take a glass of water before raiding the chocolate biscuits. It might do the trick.

How much water should you drink?

Your lifestyle, where and how you live, your diet, your age, and your exercise regime all influence your need for water. Dehydration becomes more of an issue with age, as our sense of thirst tends to weaken. The US Institute of Medicine recommends that men get about 125 ounces of water daily and that women get 91 ounces; that's about 2.5 litres.

Don't panic. That includes water from all foods and beverages. On average, we obtain about 20 per cent of our daily water from food, especially fruit and veg. (Apples are about 84 per cent water, bananas 74 per cent, and broccoli 91 per cent.) Processed food doesn't count. It is full of salt and sugar, and both of these things dehydrate.

I work on a basis of two litres of water a day; you can include herbal teas in this, as well as broth (remember that soup at night?). Strong tea, coffee, and booze don't count, since they are diuretic (they make you urinate more) and, therefore, dehydrate. Juices and sodas with high levels of sugar don't count either, as the body needs even more water to dilute the sugar concentration.

How can you tell if you are hydrated?

Don't rely on thirst alone. In fact, if you're thirsty, it's too late; you are probably already dehydrated. As ever, prevention is better than a cure. Other signs are fatigue, flushed skin, and faster breathing and pulse rate, leading to weakness, dizziness, and laboured breathing. An easy way is to check the colour of your urine. The darker your urine, the less hydrated you are. Except perhaps first thing in the morning, your urine should be light, clear or pale, like a young unoaked Sauvignon Blanc. If you think you're becoming dehydrated, move to a cool place and rehydrate, slowly, as drinking too fast can stimulate urination, resulting in—you guessed it—less hydration.

How can you drink more water?

Here's a really easy rule of thumb. *One glass of wine, one glass of water*:

- Helps keep you hydrated
- Fills your stomach
- Quenches your thirst so you drink less alcohol, as you will drink more slowly

Also, having a goal you're moving toward (drinking water) rather than one you're moving away from (drinking less alcohol) can seem much more manageable. Remember positive goal setting? It will also help you gauge how much you've had, how drunk you are, and whether or not you should stop. To a certain extent, drinking water before bed after a night out can also prevent a hangover. (See below.)

When should you drink water?

I've already suggested a large glass of room temperature water upon waking to help activate the internal organs, kick-starting the system and compensating for night-time dehydration from sweating. Try to drink water before you do just about anything—a glass of water before an alcoholic drink, a glass of water thirty minutes before a meal, and drink at least two hours before exercise. Basically, drink water. It's one of those habits we should be developing. Drinking water before eating or drinking alcohol helps start enzyme activity, which aids digestion. This idea works for coffee too, as you should always drink water with your espresso. The Italians usually serve a small glass of water with their coffee. Try and ditch milky coffee if you can; it reduces the acidity of the coffee, rendering it less digestible and adds on the calories. If you order a milky coffee after a meal in France, they'll joke about you having a late breakfast.

Try not to drink a lot of water with your meal, or a lot of wine, come to that. It slows down digestion by diluting stomach acids and enzymes and speeds up the movement of food from the stomach to the small intestine. During a conference at a detox resort, a doctor was explaining how bad it was to consume a lot of water with meals. "What about wine?" I asked. Her response was, "Well, you only drink a small amount of wine with food, so it's okay." (She has obviously never been to any of our dinner parties!)

Being hydrated before you go to bed can help avoid night-time leg cramps. Dehydration depletes the body of minerals such as magnesium, which can cause cramping. Alcohol also tends to make the body more acid. In an effort to balance its acidity, the body will use up both magnesium and calcium (often from bones) contributing to cramping. So drink water, before, during, and after drinking, and eat dark chocolate, a great source of magnesium. Red wine and chocolate is a match made in heaven and not just because of the way it tastes.

I remember complaining of leg cramps in an early-morning Pilates class. The teacher looked me in the eye and asked, "How much champagne did you drink last night?" I was stunned. He was right. Booze dehydrates, remember? I've learnt my lesson.

Waking up with achy joints after a night on the tiles is less due to alcohol itself than to dehydration. Ligaments between bones contain a lot of water to keep them soft. When they dry out, they no longer cushion the bones in the joints, causing pain.

One of the reasons people cut back on consuming water before bed, especially as they get older, is fear of needing to get up and urinate in the night. Gravity holds water in the lower part of your body when you are upright (legs swell). When you lie down and the legs are level with the kidneys, it becomes easier for the kidneys to remove the water, hence the need to urinate at night. Sorry, there's not much we can do here except reduce late afternoon diuretics (tea and coffee, as mentioned earlier).

Try and get used to drinking water at room temperature. If you find this difficult, try adding a squeeze of lemon. Drinking (and eating) things that are very cold hinders digestion. The theory that drinking icy water burns calories is negligible. If you want a healthy effect from cold water, try a cold blast in the shower before you dry off. It's brilliant for your skin and circulation and apparently encourages the percentage of fast-burning brown fat over white fat that hangs around. It's a great way to wake up, even if it does take a bit of courage first thing in the morning.

THE KISS PRINCIPLES FOR A DAILY DETOX

- Start the day with a stretch and glass of water.
- Oil pull and body brush.
- Lemon in hot water (with ginger, turmeric, and pepper for the brave).
- End the day with an early supper (no raw after four) and a ten-hour fast to ensure you get your beauty sleep.
- Drink two litres of water a day.
- Drink water before you eat, drink alcohol or coffee, or exercise.
- One glass of water, one glass of wine, repeat.
- Drink still water at room temperature.

CHAPTER SIX

THE BITTER TRUTH

Let food be thy medicine and medicine be thy food.
—Hippocrates

THIS IS NOT a classic diet book. The title could be considered a little misleading (but it is a great title). There's no calorie counting and no gorgeous recipe photos with impossible-to-source ingredients (although that might be a project for a future book).

DRINKING: A WEIGHTY MATTER

Many of us struggle with our weight so the calorie content of wine is a valid concern. Calories in wine vary depending on the style, alcohol content, and any residual sugar. A 175 ml glass of wine with 13 per cent ABV is about 160 calories. Of course sugar levels depend on the type of booze and cocktail mixer. Pure alcohol has a higher number of calories per gram than sugar, seven calories as compared to four.

There's an online calorie counter at www.drinkaware.co.uk. [53]

As if alcohol wasn't fattening enough, it also gives us the munchies. You know how you can't resist food after a few drinks? It's not just the aperitif effect on the palate that makes your mouth water; according to recent research alcohol, in the bloodstream makes the brain more sensitive to food smells.[54] That and the fact that willpower goes out the window after a few drinks means resistance to that pizza is going to be a whole lot lower! And don't tell yourself you're eating to soak up the booze. It's too late. The slowing down of alcohol absorption comes from eating before and from drinking with food. After the damage is done, it's too late.

If you are drinking with your waistline in mind, avoid sugary cocktail mixers; fruit juice with high fructose corn syrup; and Red Bull, cola, and other sodas. They are just as hard for your body to process as the alcohol, as are artificially sweetened mixers. We are trying to give our liver a break here. Try sparkling water and fresh fruit juice (no sugar added). A white wine spritzer (mineral water, not lemonade) is a great way to start a summer's evening.

Now let's talk about what we can include in our diet to improve our digestive and liver function.

EAT YOUR GREENS

A diet that includes plenty of fresh fruits and vegetables is essential for good digestive health, especially green leafy vegetables, and the bitter ones at that. Fruit and veg are not only for digestive health; the risk of having a stroke is 20 per cent to 30 per cent lower for people who eat more than five servings of fruit and vegetables a day.[55] Vitamin C found in fruit and veg is key in protecting us against infection and, it appears, cancer. Fewer than two portions of fruit and veg a day, and you are not getting your necessary daily dose.

A plant-based diet with a diversity of mainly green leafy veg, the bitterer the better, will increase your well-being.

We know that six, eight, or ten portions (depending on who you listen to) of vegetables a day are important. I say vegetables, as most fruit tends to be sugar rich, although the fibre content of whole fruits slows down the absorption of sugar. Don't eliminate fruit altogether (wine is made from grapes, after all). But concentrate on the veg and add in the fruit as an afterthought.

"My glass of wine is one of my five a day." Very funny. Wine does come from fruit. And those dietary recommendations for fruit and vegetables are due to the benefits of fibre, vitamins, and minerals but also the polyphenols, which are found in wine. It still doesn't count as one of your five a day.

Prepare to be amazed by the other treasures the plant world holds for our health.

WHICH VEG?

Alongside the vitamins, minerals, antioxidants, and fibre, plants also have "magic" ingredients called polyphenols. Plants have developed polyphenols as protection against predators, as a stress response system. The theory is that, if we ingest these elements, they, in turn, stimulate our stress response.

What's a polyphenol?

Phenolic acids—tannins, anthocyanins, procyanidins, flavanols, quercetin, and resveratrol are all terms for polyphenols found in red wine. Grapes, mainly the skin and the seeds, are a very good source.

Polyphenols are produced as a microbial defence by plants when diseases attack them. This can result in harsh and bitter flavours. Don't think only grapes from hot sunny climates have high levels of polyphenols. A longer, slower ripening period allows complexity to build in the skins, thanks to these polyphenols. This is perfect for the winemaker, who is looking for great colour, flavours, and mouth feel. Grapes from cooler, damper climates are frequently attacked by mildew, which encourages this. It's a win-win—great wine with a higher concentration of healthy polyphenols. Bordeaux, with its cooler, damp, and cloudy climate, may well be one of the best places to grow grapes with high polyphenol levels.

TOO GOOD TO BE TRUE.

The Sirtfood diet[56] hit the headlines with its claims that a glass of wine can replace an hour in the gym. Don't kid yourself. Like most things, if it sounds too good to be true, it probably is. The theory is based on SIRT xenohormesis, the biological phenomenon enabling humans to benefit from the stress responses of plants by consuming the polyphenols plants produce under stress.[57] These polyphenols are thought to produce similar effects to exercise and calorie restriction, both of which have anti-ageing effects. You might find the peppery flavour of rocket delicious, but it is designed as the plant's natural defence against being eaten by bugs.

Guess what was the sirtfood that started all this? Resveratrol, a polyphenol found in red wine.

The polyphenols trigger sirtuin genes. The authors of *The SirtFood Diet*,

Aidan Goggins and Glen Matten, (who also wrote *The Health Delusion*[58]) call these skinny genes, as they are considered metabolic regulators that encourage fat burning. Not all fat is created equal; white fat hangs around on the hips and tummy, but brown fat is easier to burn off. The theory is these sirtuins transform white fat into to brown (or beige) fat. We all have this brown or "good" fat at birth, but thanks to our high-sugar, low-activity lifestyles switching off these genes, it declines through the years and is replaced by white fat. Fasting triggers these genes. Exercise triggers them too. That's for the next chapter.

So, what are these trigger sirt foods? Everything bitter, from extra virgin olive oil to kale, parsley, rocket or arugula (also considered an aphrodisiac) to walnuts, green tea, cocoa, and turmeric. I love this concept, as all these foods are already firmly ensconced in my diet. I work well on the principle that what I love is good for me.

Some research suggests that this fat conversion happens at night, so drinking a glass of red wine in the evening might be beneficial. More seriously, it might also go some way to explaining why unhealthy sleep patterns are linked to weight gain.

A glass or two of red wine a day will not give you enough resveratrol to do the job. If you want to stock up on sirtuin activators, you need to eat your veg as well. (I told you it was too good to be true.)

A BITTER PILL

Bitter herbs and vegetables can stimulate and even help regenerate the liver (see chapter three). Foods that help your liver function are known as choleretic. The world "choleric" also means short-tempered. Your liver function is closely linked to your humour. Sound familiar?

In her brilliant book *Bitter: A Taste of the World's Most Dangerous Flavor*, Jennifer McLagan explains the role bitter plays on our palates, in our culture, and in our digestion.[59] She describes it as dangerous, indicating the possible presence of poison, with the bitterness stimulating the liver to process or rid the body of the potential toxin. Babies and young children, who have more taste buds than adults, are particularly susceptible to bitterness, which is why you might struggle to get them to eat certain greens and why coffee is an acquired adult taste. Small, young bodies are at much more risk from bitter poisons than a larger adult body, so their increased sensitivity to bitterness makes sense. It's not only children; some adults are averse to bitterness. In a taste test, it's the key element in deciding how sensitive your palate is.

Don't be too masochistic. In excess, bitterness can still be poison. Bitterness tends to be picked up at the back of the tongue or the entrance to the throat and can activate a gagging reflex, encouraging us to spit out unwanted or dangerous toxins.

Bitter foods stimulate taste receptors on the tongue, stimulating enzyme production and bile flow, which breaks fat up into smaller droplets that are easier to digest. Now you know why those bitter aperitifs make the juices flow and whet your appetite. Bitter foods also contain sulphur-based compounds, which support the natural detoxification pathways in the liver. All of a sudden that glass of tannic red wine with a steak marbled with fat makes so much sense, as does the French salad of bitter curly endives with chicken livers.

We don't eat as much bitter food in our diet as we used to. Our palates are becoming used to sweetness. Consider grapefruit. Yellow grapefruit are bitter, thanks to naringin, an antioxidant and anticancer chemical. But you'll struggle to find them now, replaced on supermarket shelves by the sweet pink grapefruit. I'm lucky enough to spend part of the year in Mauritius where "brindilles," small aubergines (eggplant), are a major ingredient. They are really bitter, much more so than the big varieties we get in Europe, where food has been bred to suit our Western palettes.

Break away. Think bitter greens and consider the initial taste shock of bitter foods to be positive, rather than negative. Bitter equals healthful. Move away from sweet to bitter—dark green veg, kale, dark chocolate, green tea, bitter olive oil, etc.

TURN TOWARDS THE TANNIC

Bitter herbs and vegetables include nettles, dandelion, horseradish, watercress, parsley, radish, milk thistle, coriander leaves, rocket, endives or chicory, and many more.

Other foods known for their choleretic benefits include artichokes (see below), turmeric, and chamomile. These contain classes of chemical such as alkaloids, terpenes, flavonoids, phenols, saponins, catechins, isothiocyanates, and other magical polyphenols that all bring benefits.

Bitterness can also stop us overeating. Unlike sugar, acidity, and fat that make your mouth water, bitterness makes you pucker up. That's why it's easier to stop after one square of dark chocolate, but you tend to munch your way through a whole bar of milk chocolate. And it's why an espresso closes your appetite at the end of a meal. See chapter four, "How to Drink Like a French Woman".

As bitterness stimulates gastric juices, "bitters" are often included in pre-dinner drinks. Think Aperol Spritz, Pink gin or Lillet, a Bordeaux wine-based aperitif with quinine bark and bitter oranges. There is even an Italian vermouth called Cynar that has artichoke extract. After-dinner drinks can be bitter too, designed for times of excess. Fernet Branca anyone? According to McLagan, a lager has more antioxidants than a glass of red wine or a cup of green tea.[1]

CRUCIFEROUS VEG

Another class of veggies we should include in our diet are brassicas. These include cabbage, Brussels sprouts, kale, swede, broccoli, mustard, horseradish, and rocket. They contain a chemical called glucosinolate, which breaks down into sulforaphane, where the sulphur smell comes from when overcooked. It helps detoxify the body by activating liver detox enzymes and may also help fight cancer. Vegetables like spinach, cos lettuce, kale, and broccoli are also excellent sources of folic acid, magnesium, and vitamins B6 and C. Spinach and parsley also contain glutamine, important for helping sleep regulation, as well as detox. Vegetable soup as a nightcap perhaps?

You can see there are a few names of veg that come up again and again in the various research data. These are the super veggies that should definitely be in your Drinking Woman's Diet. But monotony leads to boredom, and you won't stick to it. So mix it up. Variety is the spice of life.

Talking of spice, bitter spices such as turmeric with a dash of pepper can make these veggies taste a lot more interesting and add an extra dose of antioxidants.

---

[1] If you lack inspiration for how to incorporate bitter in your diet, you can follow some of the inspirational recipes from McLagen's book.

LES ARTICHAUTS DE MACAU

When matching food and wine, one vegetable that always gets bad press is the artichoke, especially with red wines. This relation of the thistle makes red wines taste metallic and tannic—not in a good way. So imagine my surprise when I first toured the Medoc, the region of Bordeaux known for some of the most famous Cabernet-driven wines of the area, to discover it is known for its artichokes too. "Les Artichauts de Macau," are a regional specialty that come from a village in the South of the Medoc (not off the south coast of China). *Strange*, I thought. That is until someone explained to me that artichokes are considered a liver tonic, which goes a long way to explaining their local popularity—especially as they are at their best in the spring, offering a spring-clean for the liver. The French are champions of seasonal eating.

ANTIOXIDANTS

In his book *The Wine Diet* (another great title), Dr Roger Corder also examines the health claims of polyphenols, concentrating on wine as a source.[60] He is a bigger fan of procyanidins (another polyphenol) than the better-known resveratrol (thanks to the French Paradox[61]). His research looked into the beneficial effects on blood circulation and heart disease, not really for weight loss or detoxification, but we'll take it. We are only as old as our arteries, after all. Procyanidins are not just in red wine of course. They're found in pine bark (sounds yummy) and cocoa (that's more like it), as well as many of the vegetables mentioned above and dark red fruits, such as cranberries and blueberries.

I mentioned procyanidins in the chapter on the liver's little helpers. These antioxidants, discovered in Bordeaux by Dr Messelier, are extracted from grape skins and pips, as well as pine bark, to make up one of the supplements I take on a regular basis.

In case you're not convinced, there's another reason to eat your greens.

PROBIOTICS AND PREBIOTICS

As well as supplying all these wonderful vitamins, antioxidants and polyphenols, vegetables are good for our digestion. Fibre in fruit and veg has long been known to be good for us, considered a bulking agent helping peristalsis (the rhythmic pressure the gut uses to push food through the system). The current recommendation is a minimum twenty-five grams of fibre per day to maintain a healthy digestive system. Fibre-rich foods include whole grains, apples, figs, pears, spinach, cruciferous vegetables, beans, and broccoli.

Fibre has a much more interesting function than just keeping us regular through mechanics. These fibres are prebiotics that feed our resident bugs, our gut microbiome—the mix of bacteria that live in the lower gut and help digest foods, expel toxins, and make up the majority of our immune system.

We talked about the importance of this microbiome in chapter three. They are important in warding off infection; decide exactly how much energy we can extract from our food; and bulk up the content of the gut, keeping us regular. Poor digestion and malabsorption creates inflammation that affects the entire body, so the effect of reduced inflammation in the gut is felt rapidly throughout the whole body.

The key to a happy healthy gut biome is to cultivate a variety of bacteria and keep them happy by feeding them what they love. They really don't like alcohol[62] (apart from an occasional glass of good red wine). Nor do they like junk food or the artificial sweeteners, emulsifiers, and preservatives found in them. They don't enjoy emotional stress and can be destroyed by antibiotics.

Guess what they do love? Yep, vegetables, and the really fibrous ones—asparagus, artichokes, garlic, onions, leeks, and chicory root are favourites. Include root vegetables such as beetroots, carrots, rutabaga (swede), and parsnips. Sulphurous veggies, such as leeks and garlic, are also top of their list. These prebiotics all contain a soluble fibre, inulin, that feeds the good bacteria, which in turn reduces the amount of toxins produced in the gut, reducing the workload of the liver.

The fibrous stalks of vegetables can be included in soups, as they will remain undigested until they reach the colon, offering a feast for your bugs. They quite like green tea, dark chocolate, a little red wine, extra virgin olive oil, dark black cherries, blueberries, and raspberries for the polyphenols.

Where do these bugs come from? They come from our mothers' birth canals, through breastfeeding, and from our diet. Include fermented foods—yoghurt, kefir, sauerkraut, raw cheese, kimchi, miso, and apple cider vinegar—in your diet. Over-the-counter supplements are also good sources, but get some advice: Not all supplements contain active bacteria, and they can also contain different concentrations and different strains. There is some question as to whether taking them orally is efficient, as they may not survive through the digestive system. There may be some truth to the old wives' tale—you have to eat a little dirt before you die. Living in too sterile an environment may be hindering the proliferation of healthy gut bacteria.

Eliminating, or at least dealing with, stress can help too. Yoga and meditation are great (see chapter seven). I mentioned fasting in the daily detox; it also helps the bacteria, giving them a break from digesting so they reproduce and work on repairing and keeping our guts healthy and strong.

In addition to all these advantages, eating more veg seems to have a positive effect on hypertension and weight gain. If you're eating all this veg, there is no time and no room on the plate left for anything fattening! However, if you are not already eating your greens, make changes to your diet slowly and keep drinking enough water to prevent gas, bloating, and stomach cramps as your body adapts to its new regime.

In a 2015 study from Chicago's Rush University Medical Center, researchers showed that following a specific *plant-heavy diet*—one that includes moderate consumption of wine—could *slow* cognitive decline in older adults with Alzheimer's or dementia.[63] Now in all this, there are a lot of maybes. It is early days for a lot of this research, but it's fascinating stuff.

FAT

Fat is good for us. Essential fatty acids are needed for the brain, immunity, and the quality of your skin. But not all fats are created equal. The demonisation of fat in recent years, with the objective of protecting us from cardiovascular disease, has only increased the obesity epidemic and all the health horrors associated with it, from diabetes to heart disease. Why? As manufacturers cut out fat to appease this trend, they replaced it with sugar, to make the foods palatable. Disaster. This has increased our consumption of sugar—one of the reasons behind the obesity epidemic. Sugar is not only fattening, it also causes inflammation leading to disease. And as we have seen above, excess sugar overloads the liver.

Which fats should we eat? We have looked at supplements in chapter three. We're looking for omega-3 and omega-6 fats, found mainly in cold-pressed vegetable oils and fatty fish. The omega-3 fatty acids, such as EPA and DHA, are the trickier ones to get hold of. Omega-3s are anti-inflammatory, can help reduce irritable bowel syndrome, and support immune function. And fat content might help protect against the damaging effects of alcohol intake if consumed before you start drinking. Remember that full fat yoghurt I mentioned earlier? Perfect before you go out for drinks if you're unsure food will be available.

Fish oils are the classic source, including wild-caught fatty fish; lake fish such as trout and smaller fatty fish such as mackerel are best. Larger fish from higher up the food chain have had bad press because of pollution, mainly from heavy metals that can become concentrated. To reduce the risk of heavy metal contamination, check your sources of both supplements and fresh fish. Trout from fresh water may be a less polluted source than salmon. Oily fish is also a great source of vitamin D.

Whose mother didn't make them swallow cod liver oil as a child? Mine still does when I go to visit, disguising it in orange juice so she thinks I won't notice. Old habits die hard. But with beautiful skin at the age of ninety, she could be on to something!

Vegetarian omega supplements tend to come from seaweed or vegetable sources, such as micro-algae, spirulina, linseed, chia, flaxseed, and walnut oils. Always keep cold-pressed oils in the fridge to reduce oxidation. Flax seeds are a great source of fatty acids; mill them first, though, to make the acids easier to get to, and keep them in the fridge small batch by small batch in case they go rancid (not good).

Some animal fats contain omega-3s. Just like we choose our wines for quality over quantity, we should use the same technique for animal fats. You don't need much, so you can afford to be picky. Free-range animals grazing outside on grass and herbs will have omega-3s in their fat, absorbed from the vegetation. Look for omega-3, free-range enriched eggs, which means that chickens had flax in their diet.

Just when you thought you couldn't eat another vegetable, you'll be happy to know some vegetables contain omegas too. Purslane, which is a weed used in Greek and Middle Eastern cookery, is a great source. If you struggle to find it (and I did say I wouldn't include weird, tricky-to-find ingredients, didn't I?), lambs lettuce (corn lettuce, mache, or nussler, depending where you live) is also a good source. Other vegetable sources of omega-3 include raw nuts and seeds, such as chia, linseed, walnuts; soybeans and their oils; and rapeseed, hemp, and flax. Chocolate has good fats too; it is a fruit, after all, and boasts oleic acid, also found in avocados, which helps lower cholesterol too.

As fat helps absorb the fat-soluble vitamins from all those veg you are eating, drizzle some cold-pressed oils on your veggies and salads, and you're good to go. Walnut oil is particularly delicious in vinaigrette. A little further east of us, in the Dordogne, walnuts are a local speciality, and they even make a bitter liqueur from them.

There is also some research that show eating fats may reduce the damage alcohol does to the liver.[64]

BURNING AND BBQS

Don't cook with cold-pressed vegetable oils, such as sunflower and corn oil, as they can break down with heat and become aldehydes, thought to be a cause of cancer. I also mentioned trans fats in the liver chapter—nasty stuff. Cook with clarified butter or ghee (removing the salt and water means it doesn't burn) or coconut oil, which also has a high smoking point.

THE CARB CONUNDRUM

I did say we were concentrating on what we can eat rather than what we can't. Nevertheless, "Don't eat the bread!" is one of the first tips I give to people joining me on wine tours if they don't want to pile on the pounds. I've said it so many times that I almost titled this book *Don't Eat the Bread*. In France, great bread is everywhere, and I don't suggest you never eat it—that would be impossible. On wine tours, after visiting cold cellars, tasting often young and tannic (bitter?) wines that stimulate the digestive juices, we sit down to lunch or dinner starving. Then, the waiter puts a basket of delicious fresh bread in front of us, and everyone dives in. Before you've even tasted the wine, one or two pieces, possibly dipped in some of that bitter olive oil or smothered in lovely salted butter, have disappeared; it doesn't touch the sides. That's a big burst of carbs (sugar) before the lovely salad, soup, or starter even arrives. You'll be full of delicious but empty calories before you even get to the cheese or dessert course.

Let's talk about French bread—those fresh baguettes, the morning croissants. When I first moved to France, I got into the habit of spreading mustard on the baguette while waiting for my steak. No wonder I put on two stone! French bread does have a saving grace; real French bread is proved slowly. The slow fermentation by yeast "digests" some of the sugars and also the gluten. So it is considerably healthier than industrial bread, for which the proving process is accelerated. Real French baguettes are inedible the next day, due to a lack of the preservatives you find in industrial bread. So if you have to weaken, France is the place to do so.

I'm aware that there are only so many calories I can eat in a day. And just as I try to ration myself to two glasses of wine a day, I am picky where those calories come from. Bread doesn't often make it, but when it does, I choose carefully. I try and find sourdough bread, as it is proved very slowly, usually with a yoghurt-based ferment rather than yeast, to convert the gluten and sugars. Or try and find bread made with organic flour or ancient grains such as quinoa, amaranth, sorghum, spelt, and millet, which are becoming more popular. Have you ever wondered why more and more people seem to be gluten intolerant?[2] One school of thought is that modern wheat has been bred to contain a lot more gluten than traditional grains, as it's easier and quicker to prove and retains more elasticity in industrial production conditions. There is another theory that weed killers, used late in industrial wheat growing to make harvesting easier, may remain as residue in flour, another argument for being aware of where ingredients in your food come from.[65]

Not all carbs are created equal. Try and avoid anything white (bread, rice, pasta, mashed potatoes). Don't eat white food is a good KISS principle. White foods have a high glycaemic load, or glycaemic index. This means that they are rapidly transformed into sugar and quickly absorbed into the bloodstream, causing a spike in sugar and insulin levels. Complex carbohydrates—whole grains, sweet potatoes, and the like—take longer to transform into simple sugars, putting less strain on the body to produce insulin and causing less inflammation and strain on the pancreas and liver. They also contain prebiotics for our gut biome to feast on.

I try and keep any resolutions simple, so they are easy to remember and easier to stick to. So if you are trying to lose some weight, alongside don't eat the bread, I would add, "No carbs after noon." Simple. A big bowl of pasta last thing at night may seem like a good idea, especially if you've had a few drinks (no willpower, "it'll soak up the booze"). We've had that conversation already. Remember, it's too late by then! It's also easy if we're feeling a little tired and lazy late in the day. Please don't. Carbs late at night, and off you go to bed full, with your digestive system struggling. As well as eating as early as possible in the evening, try to reduce the carbs on the menu.

If it is a "can't be bothered, too tired after work" issue, I sympathise. Think ahead. Stock up on other stuff that's easy to prepare. We've seen soups

---

[2] I'm not talking about Coeliac disease, which is a nasty condition, but intolerance.

are a winner—easy to digest and prepare. Make soup in batches and defrost as needed. Plus, as we've seen, many green veg have sleep-enhancing properties. It's a no-brainer.

PROCESSED MEATS

Processed meats are something else I suggest you avoid. They contain lots of chemical preservatives and nitrates. If you are going to have some, choose the best quality you can, or make your own pâté, and eat small quantities.

DON'T EAT TOO LATE IN THE DAY

Digestion is exhausting. The energy needed and the heat produced will not help you get that restorative night's sleep. The digestive system is more sluggish late in the day. Undigested protein passing through the system into the gut will then be attacked by gut flora or bacteria, producing bloating and fermentation. The toxins produced may be absorbed rather than expelled, especially if the liver is already struggling with an overload of alcohol and fats. We have talked about the daily detox and the daily fast. Breakfast like a king, lunch like a prince, and dine like a pauper may be an old wives' saying, but it's also a really good game plan. Old wives do tend to know a thing or two, speaking as one!

Don't force yourself to eat if you're not hungry, and don't be constrained by timing or boredom or social pressure. Instead, pay attention to how you really feel. Mindfulness, remember? It works for food as well as booze.

You will sleep better on an empty tummy, with a cool liver, and you'll wake up hungry, ready to breakfast like a king and start a new day of your liver-friendly life.

STRESS

Don't eat when stressed. Energy is taken away from the digestive system during times of stress. Easier said than done. What do you reach for when stressed? Wine? Chocolate? Thought so. Me too.

COOK YOUR FOOD

I know there is a big raw food movement, and I get the enthusiasm. I love a salad, and most of my lunches are salad-based when I have the choice. But raw veg are not the easiest thing to digest, despite what raw food fans will have you believe. The older you get, the more difficult it becomes. The key, at any age, is not to eat raw veggies late at night. Concentrate your salads and raw fruit in the morning and at lunch.

AND TO DRINK WITH THAT?

A simple way to cut your calorie intake is to avoid high-fat, high-sugar drinks. We often don't think about the calorie intake in what we drink. Swap your latte for black coffee and your sugar-filled fizzy drink for water with a squeeze of lemon or lime. The citrus will stop your insulin levels spiking and curb your body's tendency to store calories as fat.

Don't replace sugary drinks with low-sugar alternatives containing artificial sweeteners. They might not have sugar in them, so you think they are "slimming"; think again. When you put them in your mouth, your body thinks it's getting sugar. The brain sends that message to the body, which then produces insulin; this may lead to problems. Constantly consuming artificial sweeteners can change your palate, making you crave more sugar, and they also seem to have a negative effect on gut biome.[66] Most sweeteners are chemicals; some may even be carcinogenic.[67] What is sure is the chemical load puts another strain on the liver, which has to get rid of them.

If you are looking for something thirst-quenching, sweet or artificially sweetened drinks will not do the job. On the contrary, they will make you feel even thirstier. The same goes for tea and coffee, by the way, even unsweetened, as they are diuretics (different story).

TEA

Tea, especially green or white, is great for our skin and for our general health, with minimal caffeine and maximum flavonoids (catechins, a common group of polyphenolic compounds). A twelve-week placebo-controlled study confirmed that drinking green tea not only provides sun protection and increases blood flow and oxygen delivery into the skin, but can also improve skin elasticity and density, thus improving overall skin quality.[68] Prepare tea with water just off the boil to protect heat sensitive antioxidants.

GINGER

Ginger is a soothing food. It's a carminative (anti-flatulent) renowned for its digestive benefits, speeding up the digestive process, and it's good for easing nausea. Drink it as a tea (see the morning detox), and use it fresh in stir-fry dishes. Peppermint leaf and oil can also relax your stomach muscles and relieve indigestion. Try a cup of peppermint tea before bed. Other botanical bitters that help digestion include bitter lemons, marmalade, and bergamot, which sounds like a recipe for breakfast.

THE KISS DIET PRINCIPLES

- Eat your greens, the bitterer the better, liberally laced with cold-pressed oils.
- Develop a taste for fibrous and cruciferous vegetables.
- Choose brightly coloured fruit and veg.
- Steam or cook with ghee or coconut oil. No burnt fat.
- Eat fermented foods.
- Eat cooked vegetables in the evening—no raw after four.
- Choose complex carbs; skip the bread and other white foods.

CHAPTER SEVEN

GET PHYSICAL

I N THE DIET chapter, we talked about the sirtuin activators in green vegetables mimicking the effects of exercise and recent research claiming a glass of wine is equivalent to an hour in the gym.[69] Don't believe just eating your greens or drinking a glass of red is enough; physical activity has to be part of your life. If it sounds too good to be true, it probably is!

Exercise is key, not only for physical health (blood sugar and weight gain) but also for mental health—a healthy mind in a healthy body. When you exercise regularly, you release less cortisol (the stress hormone), and you will feel calmer. Exercise reduces oxidative stress and inflammation.

There's nothing like some physical activity (not even a glass of rouge) to make me feel better when I'm down in the dumps, generally feeling lethargic, or can't see the light at the end of a particular tunnel. Yoga, walking, and swimming are my go-to exercise options.

IT'S NOT JUST ABOUT THE WEIGHT

Exercise burns off calories, and it is also great for detoxing; heavy breathing and sweating help eliminate toxins, but targeted exercise can help elimination in other ways. Exercising your core muscles, through activities like pilates and yoga, massages and tones internal organs and stimulates your digestive system, helping to keep you regular.

Apart from improving circulation, toning muscle, giving a glow to your skin, and helping to shift weight, it'll keep you young and healthy. This, in turn, will ward off diseases associated with weight and reduce the risk of cardiac problems, diabetes, and even some cancers. With regular exercise, your cells will become more sensitive to insulin, stabilising blood sugar. Thirty minutes a day, five days a week is enough to benefit.

If a pill existed that did this much for us, we'd all be taking it. So what are you waiting for? Get off the couch.

MUSCLES: USE 'EM OR LOSE 'EM

Unless we maintain and improve muscle mass, we lose it at the rate of around one pound a year from the age of thirty-five. Keeping muscle tissue is vital to keeping both our body fat levels and our weight in check. Don't be dismayed if the scales go up a bit when you start exercising; muscle weighs more than fat. It's less your weight that counts and more your body fat percentage and the distribution of that body fat. I have a test pair of jeans; when I can't do them up, I know I'm in trouble. It's a much better measure than the scales. Pay attention to how you feel—mindfulness again.

Having greater muscle mass helps to slow down the usual age-related decline in our metabolism, and the extra strength helps prevent falls. Exercise may be one of the best aids to anti-ageing that there is.

MUSCLE AND ALCOHOL TOLERANCE

One of the reasons women have lower tolerances for alcohol than men is our higher body fat-to-muscle ratio. Exercise builds muscle mass at the expense of body fat. So exercise has positive long-term as well as short-term effects in helping our bodies process alcohol.

STRESS AND INFLAMMATION

Exercise is a great way to deal with stress, but it creates some of its own— good stress. We think of stress as negative. The fight-or-flight response creates damage due to the production of the stress hormone, cortisol, especially if it doesn't let up. But a little bit of physical stress can be a good thing. The liver may be the poster child for cell renewal, but all cells are destroyed and rebuilt constantly. Exercise stimulates this renewal; sustained exercise causes muscle damage, which has to be repaired. These repairs cause inflammation.

Like stress, inflammation is perceived as being bad, dangerous, and ageing. This is true of low-level, insidious inflammation that comes about through bad diet (too much sugar) and too much sitting around. This type of sustained inflammation leads to disease.

Post-exercise inflammation is more brutal and sporadic, so brutal that the body produces scavengers (white cells) to mend the muscle and solve the inflammation. As these elements are taken to the specific muscle that has been exercised, they bathe the whole body with the anti-inflammatory action. And voilà! A new younger body, rebuilt all over. These white cells also attack viruses and infections, so exercise is also thought to be good for building up immunity.

Chronic stress is bad, but small and regular bursts of exercise can trigger just enough stress to keep us young.

Exercise produces free radicals that need antioxidants to help mop them up. The polyphenols we mentioned in the diet chapter (including from wine) are antioxidants and can help with recuperation after exercise.

CELL REBIRTH: GROWING YOUNGER

Reproducing cells efficiently depends upon the health of your telomeres. The role of telomeres in anti-ageing is some of the latest exciting research in the field and a long story. Cells renew by dividing and reproducing their DNA. Eventually, this division takes its toll, and the DNA becomes damaged and incorrect information gets passed on. The damage happens from the ends of the strands of DNA. When we are young, the ends are protected by telomeres. These are slowly worn down through age and bad habits until they can no fulfil their role. In their excellent book *The Telomere Effect*, Nobel Prize winner Elizabeth Blackburn and health psychologist Elissa Epel explain the role of telomeres in much more detail, including the research that shows we can help protect them.[70] Guess how? Yep, exercise, green vegetables, and low stress. Is this formula sounding familiar yet?

WHAT TYPES OF EXERCISE?

There's no escape—being active is part of a healthy lifestyle. So what types of exercise should you incorporate into your lifestyle?

If you already have an exercise routine in your life, well done.

If you don't, what's holding you back? Time poor? Lack of skills? Lack of motivation? Some activities are easier to slip into your daily routine than others. Overdoing a workout can actually promote oxidative stress, and overtraining may even cause serious damage, so don't start a manic regime only to grind to a halt. Find what works for you, something you enjoy and go back to chapter two to look at motivation. The same techniques that can stop you reaching for a glass can get you off the couch.

WINE AND WORKOUTS

According to recent research at Canada's University of Alberta, resveratrol might also boost heart rate and increase muscle performance.[71] Jason Dyck and his team found in lab experiments that high doses of the natural compound resveratrol improved physical performance, heart function, and muscle strength. However, drinking alcohol before an exercise test to investigate angina has been shown to worsen angina and increase its severity, and excess alcohol in the system may slow down recovery time after exercise. Let's be clear, if you are hung-over, there's no way you're going to make that early morning yoga class.

Having said that, the night before you will probably have boundless energy on the dance floor and boogie the night away. Dancing is a really good way of burning up some excess alcohol, which is a good immediate source of energy. However, it does increase dehydration through sweating. So compensate by drinking more water not more booze as you get down on the dance floor or be prepared to pay the price the next morning.

MY SOLUTION: YOGA AND WALKING

Neither of these needs special kit (although we do like a cool yoga outfit) or extra expense. I can do them anywhere and anytime. That removes a few of those excuses.

Walking

Walking doesn't need much of an explanation. Get out there. Or not. Try these:

- Take the stairs instead of a lift.
- Get off the bus or underground a stop early.
- Use something (Fitbit, smartphone) to count your steps.
- Find a walking buddy. It's much more fun to catch up as you stroll, and chatting keeps you breathing—or at least helps you see how hard you find it to breathe. I belong to a group called the Walking Talkers. It does what is says on the box and gets us meeting up as well as exercising. I love it!
- Walk early evening, as it pushes "apéro" time back an hour. (See "Delayed Gratification" under "Motivation" in chapter two.)
- Buy or borrow a dog. Then you have to go out at least once a day. And the people you meet walking a dog—well, your social life will improve, too. Ask dog walkers!

Yoga: A mind and body detox

I'm a big fan of yoga, and yoga really fits the bill here. I organise wine and yoga retreats in Bordeaux. It may seem counter-intuitive to mix the two. But as you'll see, it works. A few sun salutations in the vines first thing in the morning before heading off to the vineyards is a great way to start a wine tasting day. Yoga doesn't have to be all "woo-woo" sitting around and chanting. You can build up a sweat and get your heart racing with yoga, too. Yoga is good for the brain, mind, heart, and body.

- Poses take *concentration*. Balancing poses in particular require concentration; as soon as your mind wanders, you topple.
- Yoga increases your *self-discipline, willpower, and self-control*. We have seen how important these skills are when it comes to managing drinking.
- Yoga is also about being in the moment, increasing *mindfulness*, a form of meditation in action.
- It reduces stress, which can be a trigger to reach for that glass that you don't really want (or need).

- Yoga builds *balance, strength*, and *flexibility*. Along with aerobic exercise, these are keys to optimum long-term health and ageing, whether you drink or not.
- Along with muscles, yoga allows you to target certain organs helpful for detox.
- Yoga can be aerobic. The heat build-up inside the body helps burn off toxins. It's an inside-out detox.
- Yoga is a whole body-mind practise that helps build body awareness.
- A regular yoga practise will create *accountability*. Trust me, if every morning you practise a similar routine, you'll know straight away whether you had too much to drink the night before. You'll know if you are (mis)treating your body by how hard it is to drag yourself to the mat.

ON YOUR HEAD

As well as the liver, one of the primary ways the body detoxes itself is through lymph flow (see the daily detox). Turning the body "on its head" helps stimulate the lymph, which helps the body to rid itself of accumulated impurities in the different organs, including the liver. Lymph circulation relies on muscle activity and gravity to work, unlike blood circulation, which is pumped by the heart. Inverted postures help the flow from the legs back towards your heart and also increase blood flow to the "master" gland, the pituitary, which regulates the entire endocrine system. Lymphocytes in the lymph attack foreign bacteria and viruses, and the liver is freed up to work on things like heavy metals, pesticides, and other toxins (alcohol). When the lymph and the liver work in tandem, health improves, and the risk of disease lessens.

Please don't try standing on your head, shoulder stands, or even hand stands on your own if you haven't done any in a while. You might think you can still kick up your heels and do cartwheels like you did at school, but your body might have other ideas. Headstands are particularly dangerous for the uninitiated, due to the strain and risk to the neck. Having said that, once you get the hang of doing handstands again, it is really cool; it does, indeed, take you back in time!

If you have never done yoga before or haven't for a while, I strongly recommend finding a yoga teacher before you start doing poses at home. A good teacher can warn you of contra-indications, adapt postures to your own needs, and correct any bad habits, so you get better not worse! Pay attention to your body. Challenge yourself, but never push too far. Don't compare yourself to others in a class. Yoga is not a competitive sport!

There are very many types of yoga and so many ways of teaching; you might have to shop around until you find a style that suits you. Ask friends or search online for recommendations; don't give up if the first class doesn't suit you. Try another. Be clear with the teacher when you start what you are looking for; explain what your objectives and your limitations are, but keep an open mind—you might learn something! Some classes are very energetic, while in others you just sit there and breathe for an hour. Persevere; the right teacher is out there somewhere. You don't have to commit to regular classes. I like to, as doing so keeps me on my toes, stops me getting lazy, and teaches me new poses. I look for a local yoga class when I'm travelling and have had some very interesting, and a few odd, experiences.

Yoga is such a wonderful discipline; it's a mind and body exercise. Once you learn the basics, you will be able to develop a yoga sequence you can do at home (or wherever you may be). All you need is a mat or, if you travelling, a towel laid out on the hotel carpet!

SUN SALUTATIONS

Since prevention is always better than cure, doing sun salutations every day will reduce the risk of having any digestion or liver problems. This is the regular practise that will help you measure how you feel every morning. It only takes minutes. Start with one and add on until you reach five a day.

I do sun salutations straight out of the shower, when my muscles are all nice and warm. It's a terrific start to the day. Once you start, you'll really feel it if you miss a day. I would recommend doing these before the poses below. The whole sequence should take about twenty minutes. Your mind and your body will thank you all day.

There are several different sun salutation routines. You can find them on the Internet or ask a teacher to show you (the best option). Just start with one a day. They get easier as you practise. In no time at all, you will surprise yourself as to how strong you become. I like the ashtanga sun salutation routine.

Sun salutation A

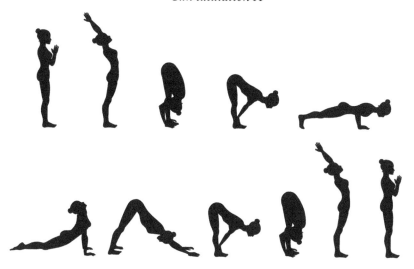

- Stand tall with feet hip's distance apart, tuck the tummy in, relax the shoulders back and down.
- Inhale and raise both arms straight above the head, looking at the hands.
- Exhale, fold forward, and look at the toes, keeping the tummy tucked in.
- Inhale and lift the spine to look straight ahead, holding on to the legs.
- Exhale, bend the knees, bring the hands to the floor on either side of the feet, and step back into a plank. Lower to the floor by bending the elbows and keeping them close to the body (it's a bit like a press-up); when you are strong you can stay hovering above the floor in chaturanga.
- Inhale, straighten the arms, and arch the back up, looking toward the ceiling, tops of the feet flat on the floor into a cobra or upward dog. (In cobra, your legs are on the floor; in upward dog, they're lifted.)
- Exhale and push back into downward dog, hips up to the ceiling, lengthening the spine and gently stretching the legs so the heels come down towards the floor. Relax the neck and gaze at your navel, with your tummy tucked in.
- Breathe deeply for five breaths.

- On the inhale, look up; step forward, bringing hands and feet together or holding the legs wherever feels comfortable. Look up.
- Exhale head down to the knees.
- Inhale—release the pressure on the knees and come all the way up, hands reached up above the head, and look up at the hands.
- Exhale back to the standing position.

Now, how good does that feel? Repeat four more times. If, after a while, that is no longer challenging enough, explore Sun Salutation B. Don't say I didn't warn you! Another advantage of a regular practise is body knowledge. If you are doing the same routine every morning, you'll soon work out when you're feeling great and not so great. It's a solid motivator for moderation the night before.

Try to introduce a little bit of movement into your morning, every morning. You'll see just fifteen, ten, or even five minutes as a regular morning habit will make a huge difference. It's not the big changes we make that affect our lives but those little, incremental, daily changes that are transformative.[3]

YOGA POSES FOR A HEALTHY LIVER

Certain postures work specifically to help massage and stimulate internal organs and digestion; some can help to stimulate the liver to function at its best. Our internal organs are made of muscle tissue, and yoga massages them, helping with blood flow and releasing tension, just as a full body massage helps the surface muscles.

You don't have to take my word for it. Alexandre Latour is an amazing yoga teacher. Trained in the discipline of ashtanga yoga,[72] he has cultivated an impressive talent for adapting yoga to individual needs and capabilities. He completely changed my approach to yoga. Here are his top five asanas (poses) for a better digestion and to stimulate the liver *(my comments in italics)*.

To be therapeutic, poses (or asanas) need to be held for a minimum of one minute to a maximum of where you are comfortable, breathing slowly and deeply and taking as few slow breaths as possible in the one-minute hold. A good range would be between one and three minutes.

Moving fast into a pose (fast vinyasa) and taking just a few breaths is

---

[3] Other resources you might like to look at are the books and videos by Beryl Bender, *Power Yoga* and *Boomer Yoga*, her personal take on the ashtanga yoga style.

less effective and not recommended when asanas are being used as a therapy (*although classes like this are a lot of fun to get the heart rate going*).

The vinyasa (movement) into all the poses are done on an exhale.

1. The wind-relieving pose *(the name is a bit of a give away!)*

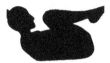

- Lie on your back with your feet together and arms beside your body.
- Breathe in and as you exhale; bring your right knee towards your chest and press the thigh on your abdomen with hands clasped around the front of the knee.
- Breathe in again, and as you exhale, lift your head and chest off the floor and try and touch your chin to your right knee. If the back of the neck starts to strain, release back to the floor.
- Hold the pose, breathing deeply and slowly in and out through the nose.
- On each exhale, tighten the grip of the hands on the knee and increase the pressure on the chest. With each inhale, loosen the grip.
- On an exhale, come back to the ground and relax.
- Repeat this pose with the left leg.
- Then repeat with both legs together.

Try rocking up and down or rolling from side to side three to five times to massage the back. Then relax.

2. The thunderbolt pose

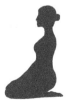

This pose is not recommended if you have knee issues.

- Kneel down, stretching your lower legs backward and keeping them together. Your big toes should cross each other.
- Gently lower your body so your buttocks are resting on your heels and the back of your thigh on your calf muscles. Gentle is the key, as this can put a lot of pressure on the knees.
- Place your hands on your knees, gazing forward with your head straight.
- Hold the pose, breathing deeply and slowly in and out through the nose.
- Closing your eyes and concentrating on your breath is very calming for the mind.

3. Spinal twist—sitting

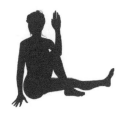

The half spinal twist is one of the best yoga postures for keeping your spine flexible and strong, soothing stiff necks and releasing upper back tension caused by stress, poor posture, or sitting too long at a desk or in front of the computer. *A flexible spine is great for holding back signs of ageing, and improved posture takes pounds off.*

It is also great for detox as the alternating compression, and release of the abdomen flushes this area with blood and massages the internal organs. *Think of old blood being squeezed out of the liver and new blood flooding back in as you release. It also tones stomach and hip muscles.*

- Sit with your legs straight out in front of you.
- Inhale and bend the left knee upward and place the left foot flat on the floor to the right (outside) of the right leg with the ankle touching the right thigh.
- Inhale and lift the right hand up, stretching up; turning the spine to the left, straighten the right arm and bring it around to the outside

of the left knee, resting against the leg and allowing some leverage to turn more.

- Turn your head as far as possible to the left and place the left hand behind your back. Keep your spine, neck, and head straight up and aligned and continue to exert effort at turning to the left. Do not compress the spine; keep lifting upwards. Breathe deeply. Do not strain the neck.
- Repeat the posture on the other side by reversing directions.

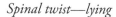

Spinal twist—lying

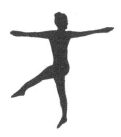

This is a relatively easy posture, done lying on the floor. Be very careful if you have disc problems. This stretches the glutes. (*The gluteus muscles are the three buttock muscles, the gluteus maximus being the largest, and we all want those nice and pert, now don't we?*) It is lovely for releasing the sciatic nerve and spine and massages those internal organs.

- Lie on the floor, arms out wide like airplane wings.
- Lift the right leg up to 90°, keeping your tummy tucked in (*might as well get a little abdominal action while we're here*).
- Bring the right leg down across the body to the left until your spine is stretched but still comfortable.
- Keep the shoulders flat on the floor.
- Look away from the leg that is across the body over your opposite right shoulder. Do not strain the neck.
- Repeat on the other side.

4. Forward bend

This posture increases the blood flow to the head (*see above for the benefits*). It also stretches the hamstrings and relieves lower back pain. It aids with digestive ailments, as folding over massages the liver, spleen, and kidneys.

Standing forward bend

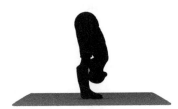

- Stand tall with feet hip distance apart, tuck the tummy in, relax the shoulders back and down.
- Bend forward from the hinge of the hips (*putting your hands on your hips will help*).
- Reach as far forward as you can, grabbing the calves, or if (when) you can, the toes.
- Let the head fall towards the floor, relax the neck and shoulders, and keep the tummy engaged.
- Allow your fingers to curl around your toes and the head to dangle in gentle traction.
- Breathe deeply through the nose.

Seated forward bend

You can also practice this one on the mat.

- Sit tall on the mat with your legs out straight in front of you.
- Tuck the tummy in and bend forward from the hinge of the hips.
- Reach as far forward as you can, grabbing the calves, or if (when) you can, the toes.

- Keep the back straight and the shoulders down and relaxed (no hunching) look at the toes to keep the neck aligned.
- Breathe deeply.

5. Triangle pose A and/or B

This is a more challenging pose that takes a while to achieve but is worth learning.

Triangle A

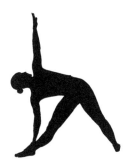

Stand like Leonardo da Vinci's *Vitruvian Man*, with feet spread across the mat making an equilateral triangle with the legs.

(You should stand like this every morning anyway. As women don't tend to own our own physical space as much as men, standing tall every morning, spreading our legs and out hands out to the sides, parallel to the floor and owning that space is as good for the mind as it is for the body. Power pose. If you don't believe me, check out Amy Cuddy's TED Talk.[73] In her research, she says woman who adopted the "Wonder Woman posture" for two minutes increased levels of testosterone by 20 per cent and decreased their stress hormone cortisol by 15 per cent.)

- Arms out to the side parallel with the mat, tummy tucked in, shoulders relaxed back and down.
- Lean to the right. *(One of my teachers used to say, vogue like Madonna; she's a yogi too.)* Keeping the body facing forwards, descend the right arm down the right leg; hold the right leg with the right hand. The objective is to reach the foot or the floor.

- When you have your balance, lift the left hand up towards the ceiling, palm facing forwards, and look up to the hand.
- If you lose your balance or your neck hurts, look back down to the floor.
- Breathe deeply for as long as you can, aiming for five inhales and exhales.
- Look down at your feet on an exhale. On the inhale, come back up, engaging the tummy muscles.
- Repeat on the left.

Triangle B

This is a little more complicated but good to learn, as it not only stimulates the liver, increases flexibility, and strengthens the legs but also exercises the brain. The cross-lateral movement forces the left and right hemispheres of the brain to work together, so it's good for brainpower too.

- Start in the same position, but this time swivel round from the left to the right.
- Bring the left hand down towards the right foot, holding the leg wherever feels comfortable. The objective is to reach the foot or the floor. If you wobble too much, come back up a little.
- Once you have your balance, bring the right hand up towards the ceiling, palm facing forwards; look up at the hand. If you lose your balance, look back down to the floor.
- Breathe deeply for as long as you can. Aim for five inhales and exhales.
- To come out, on an exhale look down at your feet. On the inhale come back up, engaging the tummy muscles.
- Repeat on the left.

So have you signed up for a yoga class yet? What are you waiting for?

AND BREATHE

Paying attention to the breath and breathing in and out through the nose, in sync with the postures, is one of the tenets of yoga. When we breathe in, our heart rate increases. When we exhale, our heart rate decreases. A longer exhalation slows our heart rate helping us to relax by activating the parasympathetic nervous system, dilating blood vessels, and creating new blood flow. It also helps stimulate the vagus nerve, which links the brain, the respiratory system, and the digestive system.

Breathing properly also helps the detox process. About 10 per cent of the alcohol leaves the body in urine, breath, and perspiration. The liver is not the only detox organ; the lungs and the skin are also important in removing toxins from the body.

"The breath of the dead" or "foetor hepaticas" is a charming name for the breath of alcoholics and binge drinkers. This peculiar sweet but fetid aroma on the breath is due to the presence of dimethyl sulphide, expelled from the blood through the lungs. Here's another motivation not to drink to excess.

Alcohol can also slow down the production of insulin by the pancreas, hindering sugar metabolism for energy, so the body burns fat instead, creating ketosis. High-protein and very low-carb diets have a similar effect. The bad breath this produces is from the by-products, ketones that build up in the bloodstream and are expelled through the lungs. All this is to show that the lungs help detox, principally removing carbon dioxide but also other compounds the body needs to get rid of from the bloodstream.

Most of us do not breath deeply enough to use the full capacity of our lungs. Yoga teaches us to pay attention to our breath, combining the breath and movement. This helps us to detox the body, but it also calms the mind, encouraging mindfulness and self-control. Remember that motivation chapter?

A SKIN-FULL

The skin, along with the gut, is the body's largest organ and plays an important role in detoxing. That sweet smell of the alcoholic can also be picked up in body odour or sweat. Alcohol in our system increases body temperature. In an effort to decrease the temperature, heart rate increases, and blood vessels dilate in the skin. This allows more blood flow to the surface of the body, releasing heat and triggering sweat glands. This process both cools the body down and helps to excrete unwanted compounds. Our bodies are very clever, if we don't let our bad habits get in the way!

Some people can suffer from skin flushing, excessive sweating, and gastrointestinal distress even at low levels of alcohol consumption due to a lack of the alcohol dehydrogenase enzyme; this situation often, but not always, affects women and people of Asian descent.

MASSAGE

Massage relieves tired muscles but can also have therapeutic uses for detoxing. This is especially true for *stomach massages*, which can help a sluggish digestive system due to a lack of regular exercise or water or vegetables.

Massage can also *stimulate the lymph* to reduce swelling, which can manifest as puffy eyelids or swollen joints. It can increase the number of white blood cells and natural killer cells. It reduces stress, which can inhibit the immune system and make you more susceptible to illness. Always drink a glass or two of water after massage to help the body flush out toxins that have been released more rapidly.

Bridget Lucas, a soft tissue therapist, who specialises in helping people invest in their own recovery, explains below the benefits of, and how to self-massage your abdomen.

SELF-MASSAGE: WHY AND HOW?

Self-massage is a highly effective way to minimise the effects of a build-up of toxins in the stomach. It stimulates and increases our blood flow, assisting lymphatic drainage, as 70 per cent of our lymph tissue resides in our gut. It relaxes the tension in the muscles around the colon, which can provide relief from constipation by stimulating the muscles required for bowel movement.

This massage will stimulate the body to release toxins through our own natural detox process, as well as providing soothing heat and comfort, aiding the release of both physical and emotional tension.

Self-massage is easiest when lying down. Ideally, allow yourself ten minutes to gain real benefit. It is the pressure you apply that increases the blood flow, whilst the circular clockwise motion of the massage will direct the flow to help release and cleanse your system.

Follow the direction of the large intestine, just above the right hip. Then, move up and across in a clockwise direction, following the way that food naturally moves and is digested.

How to self-massage

Start by lying on your back, wearing something loose fitting (or your birthday suit) and take several relaxing deep breaths.

Then begin the massage above the right hip and with one hand make several small, slow, gentle circles in a clockwise direction. Just use light pressure at this stage and create some warmth.

After about a minute, place one hand on top of the other and, again starting above the right hip, apply a light downward pressure with the heel of your hand and then release after a few seconds.

Carry on repeating this process as you work up to the right ribs, then across your stomach and down the other side, and then repeat the whole process a couple of times.

Next, apply a little more pressure with your fingertips and use slow, wavy movements, which mimic the peristalsis in the gut. Once again, begin at the right hipbone, moving up and across and then down the left side. Use enough pressure to feel an effect, but not so much that anything is painful.

Repeat the process a second time.

Finish off with some slow, gentle circular movements across the whole of the stomach.

Doing this for ten minutes a day, particularly when you've been drinking, helps your stomach and your digestive system better cope with the effects of alcohol and other toxins on your body.

COMPRESS

Along with Bridget's massage technique, we can physically help the digestive system by using a compress to help the night-time liver action. This might sound counter-intuitive if you are suffering from night sweats and palpitations that may or may not be brought on by too much alcohol overworking the liver, but bear with me.

As the liver is at its most active at about 4 a.m., we "feel the heat" as it works at a higher temperature than the rest of the body. You can help it along using a warm compress. Before you go to bed, wrap a hot water bottle in a towel and place it on the liver, just below the ribs to the right hand side of the body. This warms up the liver and encourages it to start working, helping the detox process along.

THE KISS PRINCIPLES FOR GETTING PHYSICAL

- Do thirty minutes of exercise a day, five days a week.
- Start small; be consistent.
- Find something you love.
- Remember how good it feels when you finish; that will motivate you to go back to it.
- Breathe deeply and regularly.
- Learn to self-massage the stomach to help stimulate digestion.
- Use a compress on your liver if you have had a heavy night.

A KISS GOODBYE:
SOME FINAL THOUGHTS
AND CONCLUSIONS

P ASTEUR, THE FAMOUS nineteenth-century French scientist and bacteriologist, said, "Wine is the most healthful and hygienic of all beverages." He should know; he "discovered" fermentation and inoculation!

Are there really benefits to moderate alcohol consumption? We have been looking at trying to moderate our alcohol consumption and to live a lifestyle that will hopefully compensate for the odd transgression. It's worth looking at the idea that moderate drinking may have health benefits, reducing the risk of certain diseases, especially coronary heart disease. Research shows that plotting mortality rates against drinking creates a J-shaped curve, indicating that moderate drinkers seem to live longer than teetotallers but that these benefits decline rapidly with excess.[74]

This is also known as the French paradox, a phrase coined by an American doctor in the 1980s to describe how, despite a high-fat diet, the French have lower rates of heart disease than Americans. A doctor from Bordeaux picked it up in the 1990s and attributed the difference to a moderate consumption of red wine. We now know, however, that sugar, rather than fat, is a cause of heart disease. The reputation of the health benefits of red Bordeaux has, nevertheless, not looked backed since.[75]

The counterarguments to this positive role of alcohol on health are that moderate drinkers tend to also have other positive lifestyle factors, including exercise and a healthy diet (fruit and veg) and tend not to smoke. All this together may reduce the occurrence of many chronic diseases—which is the tenet of this book!

Women in particular have been shown to benefit from moderate wine consumption. A 2015 study showed that women who engaged in six "healthy lifestyle factors," one of which was up to one drink per day on average, were significantly more likely to remain healthy over time. You can guess what the others are—not smoking, maintaining a low body mass index, engaging in at least two and a half hours of physical activity per week, watching no more than seven hours of television per week, and eating a healthy and balanced diet.[76]

THE HEART OF THE MATTER

Why these supposed benefits? A small amount of alcohol is thought to have a positive effect in stimulating the liver to produce "good" HDL cholesterol, which is anti-inflammatory. Added to this the antioxidant effects of phenols, such as resveratrol and proanthocyanidins in red wine, protect against the oxidation of LDL, the bad cholesterol.[77] So with red wine it's a double whammy. More research is being carried out to understand these mechanisms.

WHY NOT GRAPES?

Why not eat grapes or drink grape juice to get the polyphenols? It seems that the polyphenols are more bioavailable to us in wine than they are in the unfermented fruit.[78] We mentioned the benefits of alcohol above, but aside from those, it is the fermentation process that appears to make the polyphenols and antioxidants more readily available. Think about the flavours in your mouth when you chew on a grape compared to sipping a glass of wine. There is less flavour in the grape. However, if you keep the grape skins in your mouth long enough, enzymes from saliva will start to break down the skins, and the tastes will be revealed. In the wine, this work has already been for done for us. Grapes destined for wine tend to be smaller and have thicker skins than table grapes. This means a greater concentration of the polyphenols we are looking for, in terms of both pleasure and health terms.

Enzymes are released by yeast making them easier for us to absorb. Alcohol present in wine may also make these polyphenols more bioavailable Adding vodka to your cranberry juice will not do; the job has to be done during the fermentation process.

There are polyphenols in white wines too from the pulp, but in red wine the levels increase dramatically due to the maceration process (red wines sitting in the grape juice during fermentation). Winemaking techniques can also add other polyphenols to the mix. Barrel ageing of wines allows polyphenols (tannins) from the wood to be dissolved into both red and white wine as it ferments or matures in oak. Oak naturally contains high levels of polyphenols called gallotannins and vanillin, which is where the vanilla flavour in some wines comes from.

De-alcoholised red wine doesn't work as well, and it tastes disgusting.[79] More research is ongoing to discover to what extent these components are bioavailable and whether alcohol plays a role in their absorption.[80]

A meta-analysis of studies about heart heath and drinking by the Harvard School of Public Health concluded that although heavy drinking (six or more drinks in a night) increases stroke and heart attack risk, both in the short term and the long term, drinking about two drinks in a night may actually *lower* the same risks over the next week.[81] Remember our two drinks a day rule? And it would also appear that moderate drinking with meals delivers maximum health benefits. Again, wine with food.[82]

Everything seems to point to moderate alcohol consumption, preferably red wine, as part of a healthy lifestyle, including a diet rich in vegetables and regular exercise.

Having said all that, I want to make it clear that I don't drink wine (and the odd glass of gin or whisky) for the health benefits. I drink wine because I love it. I love its diversity. I love the history behind it. I love the passion of the winemakers. And I love the conviviality it brings. I can share it with friends. It makes food taste better and an evening more fun.

Moderation and drinking as part of a healthy
lifestyle are the key points to remember.
An unhealthy lifestyle watered down with the odd
glass of "rouge" will not do the job.

THE KISS PRINCIPLE

I have tried to sum up at the end of each chapter using The KISS principle: Keep It Simple Stupid. The theory being that, if things are simple, they are easier to remember and easier to implement.

Setting yourself small easy-to-attain daily goals will help you on the way to your big objectives. To sum it all up, here are some key things that work for me:

- **Drink less** – No more than two glasses a day, five days a week
- **But better** – Learn to appreciate what is in your glass and take time to enjoy it. See, smell, swirl, and sip.
- **Pay attention** to why you reach for that glass.
- **Eat first and then drink.**
- **Drink water** – two litres a day and a glass before just about everything!
- **Move** – At least thirty minutes of exercise a day, five days a week.
- **Eat your (bitter) greens**, liberally laced with good fats.
- **Don't eat the bread**; or at least be really picky about what bread you eat and when.
- **Consider taking supplements** (vitamins, minerals, antioxidants, probiotics, omega-3s).
- **Avoid other toxins**. Don't smoke, and no junk food full of additives.
- **Sleep** at least seven hours a night.
- **Detox daily**. Stretch and drink water upon waking. Drink hot lemon water thirty minutes before breakfast. Practice oil pulling and body brushing.
- Learn how to **stomach massage**.
- Keep that **liver compress** to hand.
- **Get help** if you think you have an issue with drink.
- **Enjoy your wine; enjoy your life.**

I go to bed early. I meditate. I eat all the correct foods. I don't smoke or drink, and I believe with a passion in myself. You can only beat nature when you show the bitch who's boss.
—Mae West

HOW TO SURVIVE A WINE TOUR

I T SEEMS ONLY fair to include this information, as it really was where the book started. Here are a few tips for clients joining me for a wine tour, so they don't roll onto the plane at the end of a week of wine tastings and dinners:

- Start the day with a walk or join me for fifteen minutes of sun salutations. If you're staying in the vineyard, get up a little earlier and walk out in the vines. Enjoy some fresh air and work up an appetite for breakfast.

- Eat breakfast. You might not feel like it after a big wine dinner the night before, but a full stomach (especially fats and protein) will slow down the absorption of alcohol into the bloodstream when you're tasting in the morning. Take the eggs and have some yoghurt for those probiotics.

- Take your supplements. Alcohol can be as challenging for your gut flora as for your liver, so take some probiotics alongside your milk thistle. Another excellent supplement is glutathione, which is better known in the wine trade for preserving the freshness of white wines. It might help preserve the liver, too.

- Drink a glass of water before each tasting and before eating. Keep a bottle with you to sip on throughout the day.

- Don't be shy about spitting, especially barrel samples. (And don't wear white!) It's not considered rude to the winemaker if you don't drain each glass.

- At lunch, don't eat the bread. Trickier than it sounds. When you sit down, starving after a morning of tasting, it seems impossible to resist the basket of fresh French bread on the table. But resist you must. If not, you'll never make it through lunch.

- There are not always many vegetables on offer in French restaurants. Menus often concentrate on "noble" products, such as foie gras, dismissing veggies as homely; if they do offer a vegetable accompaniment, it's usually potatoes. (There's a reason they're known as French fries.)

    In a French home, though, vegetables are key; a French family meal will usually start with either salad (crudités) in the summer or soup in the winter. Vegetables will be served with the main course and salad offered with cheese will be served before dessert.

- If there is no veg proposed with your chosen dish at a restaurant, ask to change the potatoes for the vegetable of the day or some salad. They are usually happy to oblige.

- Take a nap on the bus on the way home.

A BRIEF INTRODUCTION TO WINE TASTING

To appreciate wine, we usually go through three stages—sight, smell, and taste.

TOOLS OF THE TRADE

Wine glasses come in all shapes and sizes, and they do affect the way a wine tastes. You really don't need different wine glass shapes for different wines, although it is fun. Ideally, you'll want a clear glass with a stem; this will ensure that you can see the colour of the wine and that the heat from your hand won't warm it up. The bowl of the glass should be wider at the bottom and narrower at the top, to trap in the aromas.

WINE TASTING

Don't fill your glass too full; about one-third will do. This will allow you to swirl the wine in the glass without getting it down your shirt! Too full and you can't even get your nose in to smell the aromas of the wine.

See

Tilt the glass over a white surface, look at the colour and density, meaning how easy it is to see through it. Wine is a living, evolving thing, even when bottled. A young red wine will tend to be purple in colour and will become more ruby red and eventually tawny and brown with age. A young white wine will have greenish tinges when young, becoming more yellow and then also brownish with age if you keep it long enough.

This evolution will vary depending upon the wine. Normally, less dense wines—wines that are easier to see through—will age more quickly than deeper, darker, more purple wines. Most bottles you find on wine shop and supermarket shelves will be ready for drinking and not need ageing.

Legs, or tears, are when the wine sticks to the side of the glass. They don't really mean very much; the different ingredients of wine (water, alcohol, sugar, and so on) have different surface tensions, so they stick to the side of the glass in different ways when mixed, creating this phenomena. It's generally a sign of alcohol concentration.

Smell

Bouquet is how we describe the smell of a wine when there are lots of different aromas present. Put your nose in the glass above the wine, and you should smell anything from fruit (it's made from grapes after all!) to spices or woody notes or, in older wines, you might even smell leathery or mossy notes.

Then give your glass a swirl and smell again. Moving the glass around allows more air to come into contact with the wine and releases more aromas. It should smell stronger and perhaps more complex as more and different aromas release.

Taste

Different people are more or less sensitive to different tastes, especially bitter, which is why we all tend to like different things. Again, there is no right or wrong. Whether you like a wine or not is your personal choice. You may taste sweetness or acidity. Taste, flavour, and smell are very interwoven; try tasting with a nose clip on, and you will hardly taste anything!

But it's not just the taste. Wine has mouth feel—the sensation on the palate. Does it feel round? Soft? Smooth? Astringent? Does it leave your mouth dry or does it make your mouth water? Compare what water feels like swirling around your mouth. It's different.

Tannins are the things that give a wine body (some of the famous polyphenols we've mentioned previously). If you want to understand the difference between acid and tannins, put some lemon juice in water. That's acid. To understand what tannins feel like, leave a strong tea bag in a mug of hot water. Once it's cold, swirl it around the mouth. That's tannins. The sensations are quite different.

The *attack* of the wine, the first sensation in the mouth, is often fruity. Then mid-palate, you start to get the notion of mouth feel—acidity, grip (tannins), smoothness. The *finish* is the final sensation or impression. After that comes *length*—the length of time the flavours and sensations stay in the mouth after you have swallowed (or spat out) the wine.

Once you start paying attention to what you are drinking, taking time to smell, swirl, and taste, you will tend to drink less and possibly better. If you drink less, you can afford to drink better.

BIBLIOGRAPHY, LINKS, SOURCES AND RESOURCES

I'VE ENJOYED LOOKING up the many and various research papers into the effects of alcohol and wine, both good and bad. Some of it is frankly hilarious. You have to ask yourself, how do they come up with some of these research projects?

Some, of course, are confirming the bloody obvious; you feel like shouting, "I knew that!" But the scientific model must be respected. If you would like more details, please follow the links below.

The links to most of the research I've quoted are below.

OTHER RESOURCES AND FURTHER READING

Love your liver. Visit http://loveyourliver.org.uk (the site of the campaign of the British Liver Trust).

Feel you may have problems with alcohol? Help is at hand. Speak to your doctor or contact one of the many associations that can help. In the UK:

- Drinkline – Free, confidential, accurate, and consistent information and advice to callers who are concerned about their own or someone else's drinking. Helpline: 0300 123 1110 (weekdays 9 a.m.–8 p.m., weekends 11 a.m.–4 p.m.)
- Addiction – A UK-wide treatment agency, helping individuals, families, and communities to manage the effects of drug and alcohol misuse. Visit http://www.addaction.org.uk.

- Alcoholics Anonymous – http://www.alcoholics-anonymous.org.uk
- Al-Anon – Worldwide support and understanding for the families and friends of problem drinkers. Confidential helpline 0207 4030888 (open 10 a.m.–10 p.m.). Visit http://www.al-anonuk.org.uk.

RECOMMENDED READING

Blackburn, Elizabeth, and Epel, Elissa, *The Telomere Effect* (Orion Spring).

Bost, Brent Bost, *The Hurried Woman Syndrome* (McGraw-Hill Education).

Convile, Clare, *The Book for Dangerous Women* (Grove Press).

Corder, Roger, *The Wine Diet* (Sphere).

Edwards, Tony, *The Good News about Booze* (Premium Publishing).

Goggins, Aidan, and Hodder, Glen Matten, *The SIRT Food Diet* (Yellow Kite)

Goude, Jamie, *Wine Science: The Application of Science in Winemaking* (University of California Press)

Hamblin, James, *If Our Bodies Could Talk* (Anchor).

Matten, Glen, and Goggins, Aidan, *The Health Delusion* (Hay House UK).

McGonigal, Kelly, *The Willpower Instinct* (Avery).

McLagan, Jennifer, Bitter: *A Taste of the World's Most Dangerous Flavor* (Jacqui Small LLP).

Robbins, John, *Diet for a New America* (HJ Kramer/New World Library).

Swenson, David, *Ashtanga Yoga: The Practice Manual* (Ashtanga Yoga Productions). California Press).

ENDNOTES

1   Tim Slade, Cath Chapman, Wendy Swift, Katherine Keyes, Zoe Tonks, ad Maree Teesson, "Birth Cohort Trends in the Global Epidemiology of Alcohol Use and Alcohol-Related Harms in Men and Women: Systematic Review and " Metaregression", *BMJ Journals* (2016), http://bmjopen.bmj.com/content/6/10/e011827.

2   Thomas Atkin, Linda Nowak and Rosanna Garcia, «Women wine consumers: information search and retailing implications», International Journal of Wine Business Research (2007) https://www.sonoma.edu/users/a/atkint/forms/Atkin,%20Nowak%20and%20Garcia%20(2007)%20-%20Women%20Wone%20Consumers.pdf

3   Ibid.

4   "Alcohol a Women's health issue", National Institute on Alcohol abuse and Alcoholism: https://pubs.niaaa.nih.gov/publications/brochurewomen/women.htm

5   "Recommendations for older drinkers", National Institute on Alcohol abuse and Alcoholism: https://www.niaaa.nih.gov/alcohol-health/special-populations-co-occurring-disorders/older-adults

6   Alcohol and cancer, Drinkaware.co.uk : https://www.drinkaware.co.uk/alcohol-facts/health-effects-of-alcohol/diseases/alcohol-and-cancer/

7   Robin D. Clugston and William S. Blaner, "The Adverse Effects of Alcohol on Vitamin A Metabolism": http://www.ncbi.nlm.nih.gov/pmc/articles/PMC3367262/

8   Kelly E. Courtney and John Polich, Binge Drinking in Young Adults: Data, Definitions, and Determinants: https://www.ncbi.nlm.nih.gov/pmc/articles/PMC2748736/

9   James Hamblin, *If Our Bodies Could Talk: A Guide to Operating and Maintaining a Human Body* (New York, 2016).

10 Feskanich D, Korrick SA, Greenspan SL, Rosen HN, Colditz GA, "Moderate alcohol consumption and bone density among postmenopausal women" : https://www.ncbi.nlm.nih.gov/pubmed/10094083 J Womens Health 1999

11 WHO report on Alcohol & violence: http://www.who.int/violence_injury_prevention/violence/world_report/factsheets/fs_intimate.pdf

12 University of Bristol, Tobacco and Alcohol Research group, "**Attractiveness increases after one drink, but no more**" http://www.bris.ac.uk/expsych/research/brain/targ/news/2015/attractiveness-increases-after-one-drink-but-no-more.html

13 William H. George, Kelly Cue Davis, Julia R. Heiman, Jeanette Norris, Susan A. Stoner, Rebecca L. Schacht, Christian S. Hendershot, and Kelly F. Kajumulo "Women's Sexual Arousal: Effects of High Alcohol Dosages and Self-Control Instructions" https://www.ncbi.nlm.nih.gov/pmc/articles/PMC3159513/

14 Jennifer O'Brien for UCSF News Center: UCSF Gallo "Scientists Show That Drinking Releases Brain Endorphins https://www.ucsf.edu/news/2012/01/11298/study-offers-clue-why-alcohol-addicting. Mondaini N, Cai T, Gontero P, Gavazzi A, Lombardi G, Boddi V, Bartoletti R. Journal of Sexual Medicine, 2009 Regular moderate intake of red wine is linked to a better women's sexual health: https://www.ncbi.nlm.nih.gov/pubmed/19627470.

15 Sharon D. JohnsonDeborah L. PhelpsLinda B. Cottler, The Association of Sexual Dysfunction and Substance Use Among a Community Epidemiological Sample, archives of Sexual Behaviour, 2004 http://link.springer.com/article/10.1023%2FB%3AASEB.0000007462.97961.5a?LI=true#page-1

16 Mondaini N1, Cai T, Gontero P, Gavazzi A, Lombardi G, Boddi V, Bartoletti R. **Regular moderate intake of red wine is linked to a better women's sexual health Journal of Sexual Medicine, 2009**: http://www.ncbi.nlm.nih.gov/pubmed/19627470

17 Public Health England, "Drinking," in *One You* (campaign), http://www.nhs.uk/Change4Life/Pages/alcohol-lower-risk-guidelines-units.aspx.

18 The British Liver Trust: https://www.britishlivertrust.org.uk.

19 Drinking and You, US Guidelines: http://www.drinkingandyou.com/site/us/moder.htm

20 Dr Adam Winstock, Dr Monica Barratt, Dr Jason Ferris & Dr Larissa Maier Global Drugs Survey: https://www.globaldrugsurvey.com/wp-content/themes/globaldrugsurvey/results/GDS2017_key-findings-report_final.pdf.

21 Abdallah K. Ally, Melanie Lovatt, Petra S. Meier, Alan Brennan, and John Holmes, "Developing a Social Practice-Based Typology of British Drinking Culture in 2009–2011: Implications for Alcohol Policy and Analysis", *Wiley Online Library* (2016), https://doi.org/10.1111/add.13397 (http://onlinelibrary.wiley.com/doi/10.1111/add.13397/abstract).

22 Office for National Statistics "Adult drinking habits in Great Britain: 2005 to 2016": https://www.ons.gov.uk/peoplepopulationandcommunity/healthandsocialcare/druguseclcoholandsmoking/bulletins/opinionsandlifestylesurveyadultdrinkinghabitsingreatbritain/2005to2016

23 The Cage Questionnaire was developed in 1968 at North Carolina Memorial Hospital to help detect problem drinking behaviors.

24 The Alcohol Use Disorders Identification Test (AUDIT) **is a 10-item screening tool developed by the World Health Organization (WHO) to assess alcohol consumption, drinking behaviors, and alcohol-related problems.** https://www.drugabuse.gov/sites/default/files/files/AUDIT.pdf.

25 A few of the resources available in the United Kingdom if you feel you need help with alcohol consumption include:

- *Drinkline* – Free, confidential, accurate, and consistent information and advice to callers who are concerned about their own or someone else's drinking. Helpline: 0300 123 1110 (weekdays 9 a.m.–8 p.m., weekends 11 a.m.–4 p.m.)
- *Addiction* – A UK-wide treatment agency, helping individuals, families, and communities to manage the effects of drug and alcohol misuse, http://www.addaction.org.uk
- *Alcoholics Anonymous* – http://www.alcoholics-anonymous.org.uk
- *Al-Anon* – Worldwide support and understanding for the families and friends of problem drinkers. Confidential Helpline 0207 4030888 (open 10 a.m.–10 p.m.), http://www.al-anonuk.org.uk

26 Jennifer O'Brien for UCSF News Center: "UCSF Gallo Scientists Show That Drinking Releases Brain Endorphins" https://www.ucsf.edu/news/2012/01/11298/study-offers-clue-why-alcohol-addicting.

27 Brent Bost, *The Hurried Woman Syndrome* (McGraw-Hill Education, 2005),

28 Emily L. Zale, Stephen A. Maisto, and Joseph W. Ditrea, «Interrelations between Pain and Alcohol: An Integrative Review» National Institute on Alcohol Abuse and Alcoholism (2013) https://pubs.niaaa.nih.gov/publications/PainFactsheet/Pain_alcohol.pdf https://www.ncbi.nlm.nih.gov/pmc/articles/PMC4385458/.

29 Clare Convile, *The Book for Dangerous Women* (Grove Press USA 2012).

30 Kelly McGonigal, *The Willpower Instinct* **How Self-Control Works, Why It Matters, and What You Can Do to Get More of It** (Avery 2011).

31 Ibid

32 Rachel Pechey, Dominique-Laurent Couturier, Gareth J. Hollands, Eleni Mantzari, Marcus R. Munafò and Theresa M. Marteau **Does wine glass size influence sales for on-site consumption? A multiple treatment reversal design** BMC Public HealthBMC (2016) https://bmcpublichealth.biomedcentral.com/articles/10.1186/s12889-016-3068-z.

33 National Institute of Neurological Disorders ad Stroke "Brain Basics: Understanding Sleep" (2017) https://www.ninds.nih.gov/Disorders/Patient-Caregiver-Education/Understanding-Sleep

34 Yuko Nakanishi, Koichi Tsuneyama, Makoto Fujimoto, Thucydides L. Salunga, Kazuhiro Nomoto, Jun-Ling An, Yasuo Takano, Seiichi Iizuka, Mitsunobu Nagata, Wataru Suzuki, Tsutomu Shimada, Masaki Aburada, Masayuki Nakano, Carlo Selmi M. Eric Gershwin, "Monosodium glutamate (MSG): A villain and promoter of liver inflammation and dysplasia" Journal of Autoimmunity (2008) https://www.sciencedirect.com/science/article/pii/S0896841107001400.

35 Elizabeth Brandon-Warner, Ph.D., Laura W. Schrum, Ph.D., C. Max Schmidt, M.D., Ph.D., and Iain H. McKillop, Ph.D.: Rodent Models of Alcoholic Liver Disease: Of Mice and Men https://www.ncbi.nlm.nih.gov/pmc/articles/PMC3496818/ (Bradford et al. 2005).

36 John Robbins, *Diet for a new America: How Your Food Choices Affect Your Health, Happiness, and the Future of Life on Earth* (HJ Kramer/New World Library 2012).

37 Lifeplus: https://lifeplus.com/wendynarby. Disclaimer: I act as a distributor for these vitamins.

38 Jason Allen, ND, MPHand Ryan D. Bradley, ND, MPH "Effects of Oral Glutathione Supplementation on Systemic Oxidative Stress Biomarkers in Human Volunteers": https://www.ncbi.nlm.nih.gov/pmc/articles/PMC3162377/.

39 Vishnudutt Purohit, J. Christian Bode, Christiane Bode, David A. Brenner, Mashkoor A. Choudhry, Frank Hamilton, Y. James Kang, Ali Keshavarzian, Radhakrishna Rao, R. Balfour Sartor, Christine Swanson, and Jerrold R. Turner «Alcohol, Intestinal Bacterial Growth, Intestinal Permeability to Endotoxin, and Medical Consequences Summary of a Symposium" https://www.ncbi.nlm.nih.gov/pmc/articles/PMC2614138/.

40 Eurostat"Proportion of overweight and of obese women" (2014): http://ec.europa.eu/eurostat/statistics-explained/index.php/File:Proportion_of_overweight_and_of_obese_women,_2014.png

41 National Institute of Diabetes and Digestive and Kidney Diseases, "**Overweight & Obesity Statistics**" https://www.niddk.nih.gov/health-information/health-statistics/overweight-obesity

42 The World Health Organisation, «Global status report on alcohol and health 2014» : http://www.who.int/substance_abuse/publications/global_alcohol_report/msb_gsr_2014_3.pdf.

43 Ibid.

44 Some of my favourite wine and food matching books:
  • Joanna Simon, *Wine with Food: The Ultimate Guide to Matching Wine with Food for Every Occasion* (London 1999)

- Michel Roux Jr, *Matching Food & Wine: Classic and Not So Classic Combinations (London 2005)*
- David Rosengarten & Joshua Wesson *Red Wine with Fish: The New Art of Matching Wine with Food* (London 1989)

45 Matthew L. Lindberg, MD and Ezra A. Amsterdam, MD, « Alcohol, Wine, and Cardiovascular Health « Division of Cardiovascular Medicine, University of California-Davis, Sacramento, California, USA (2007) https://onlinelibrary. wiley.com/doi/pdf/10.1002/clc.20263

46 Mladen Boban, Creina Stockley, Pierre-Louis Teissedre, Patrizia Restani, Ursula Fradera, Claudia Stein-Hammer and Jean-Claude Ruf «Drinking pattern of wine and effects on human health: why should we drink moderately and with meals?» food anf Function '(2016) http://pubs.rsc.org/-/content/articlepdf/2016/ fo/c6fo00218h.

47 Wine and Spirits Education Trust (WSET): https://www.wsetglobal.com.

48 **Sarah Jane Banks, Karthik Ramakrishnan Sreenivasan, David M. Weintraub, Deanna Baldock, Michael Noback, Meghan Pierce, Johannes Frasnelli, Jay James, Erik Beall, Xiaowei Zhuang, Dietmar Cordes, Gabriel C Léger" Structural and Functional MRI Differences in Master Sommeliers: A Pilot Study on Expertise in the Brain, Frontiers** in Human Neuroscience, (2016) http://journal.frontiersin.org/article/10.3389/fnhum.2016.00414/full.

49 Roger B. McDonald, and Jon J. Ramsey, Honoring Clive McCay and 75 Years of Calorie Restriction Research The Journal of Nutrition, (2010) https://www. ncbi.nlm.nih.gov/pmc/articles/PMC2884327/.

50 Lo learn more about the 5:2 Diet visit https://thefastdiet.co.uk.

51 To learn more about David F. Dinges, his work with the Center for Sleep and Circadian Neurobiology at Perelman School of Medicine, and a list of related publications, visit Dinges's faculty page at http://www.med.upenn.edu/apps/ faculty/index.php/g362/p6693.

52 To learn more about the Mayr Clinic visit: https://www.vivamayr.com/en/.

53 To see the drink aware calorie counter visit : https://www.drinkaware.co.uk/ understand-your-drinking/unit-calculator.

54 Obesity Society. "Alcohol sensitizes brain response to food aromas, increases food intake in women." ScienceDaily. ScienceDaily, 30 June 2015. www. sciencedaily.com/releases/2015/06/150630122252.htm

55 Dagfinn Aune, Edward Giovannucci, Paolo Boffetta, Lars T Fadnes, NaNa Keum, Teresa Norat, Darren C Greenwood, Elio Riboli, Lars J Vatten and Serena Tonstad. «**Fruit and vegetable intake and the risk of cardiovascular disease, total cancer and all-cause mortality—a systematic review and dose-response meta-analysis of prospective studies**» The international Journal of Epidemiology (2017) https://academic.oup.com/ije/article/46/3/1029/3039477

56 Aidan Goggins and Glen Matten *The Sirtfood Diet*, (Hodder, London 2016).

57   Philip L. Hooper, Paul L. Hooper, Michael Tytell, and László Vígh «Xenohormesis: health benefits from an eon of plant stress response evolution», Cell Stress Chaperones (2010) https://www.ncbi.nlm.nih.gov/pmc/articles/PMC3024065/.

58   Glen Matten and Aidan Goggins, *The Health Delusion* (Hay House UK 2012).

59   Jennifer McLagan, *Bitter, A Taste of the World's Most Dangerous Flavor (Ten Speed Press 2014)*.

60   Roger Corder, *The Wine Diet* (Sphere 2009).

61   Serge Renaud, a scientist from Bordeaux University is credited with coining the phrase "The French Paradox" to explain the relatively low rates of heart disease in the French populations, despite their high fat consumption. His conclusion was the polyphenol resveratrol was, at least partly, responsible. The theory became popular when it was picked up by CBS in its programme *60 Minutes* in the 1990s. See the news item here: https://youtu.be/rMNG0zbZlmE.

62   Gabbard SL1, Lacy BE, Levine GM, Crowell MD»**The impact of alcohol consumption and cholecystectomy on small intestinal bacterial overgrowth».** Department of Gastroenterology and Hepatology, Cleveland Clinic (2014) https://www.ncbi.nlm.nih.gov/pubmed/24323179.

63   Diet May Help Prevent Alzheimer's, Rush University Medical Center (2015) https://www.rush.edu/news/diet-may-help-prevent-alzheimers

64   Kirpich IA, Feng W, Wang Y, Liu Y, Barker DF, Barve SS, McClain CJ «**The type of dietary fat modulates intestinal tight junction integrity, gut permeability, and hepatic toll-like receptor expression in a mouse model of alcoholic liver disease».** Division of Gastroenterology, Hepatology, and Nutrition, Department of Medicine, University of Louisville School of Medicine, Kentucky, USA. (2012) http://www.ncbi.nlm.nih.gov/pubmed/?term=The+type+of+dietary+fat+modulates+intestinal+tight+junction+integrity%2C+gut+permeability%2C+and+hepatic+toll-like+receptor+expression+in+a+mouse+model+of+alcoholic+liver+disease.

65   Pesticide Action network UK (2014), "Pesticides in Your Daily Bread: A Consumer Guide to pesticides in Bread" http://issuu.com/pan-uk/docs/pesticides-in-your-daily-bread-2014?e=28041656/49217321.

66   Jotham Suez, Tal Korem, Gili Zilberman-Schapira, **Eran Segal** & **Eran Elinav** «**Non-caloric artificial sweeteners and the microbiome: findings and challenges»** Journal of Gut Microbes (2015) https://www.tandfonline.com/doi/full/10.1080/19490976.2015.1017700.

67   Whitehouse CR1, Boullata J, McCauley LA «**The potential toxicity of artificial sweeteners»** Adult Health/Gerontology Nurse Practitioner Program, School of Nursing, University of Pennsylvania (2008). https://www.ncbi.nlm.nih.gov/pubmed/18604921.

68   Ulrike Heinrich, Carolyn E. Moore, Silke De Spirt, Hagen Tronnier and Wilhelm Stahl «Green Tea Polyphenols Provide Photoprotection,

IncreaseMicrocirculation, and Modulate Skin Properties of Women» Journal of Nutrition (2011) http://www.beauty-review.nl/wp-content/uploads/2013/12/Green-tea-polyphenols-provide-photoprotection-increase-microcirculation-and-modulate-skin-properties-of-women.pdf.

69 Vernon W. Dolinsky Kelvin E. Jones Robinder S. Sidhu Mark Haykowsky Michael P. Czubryt Tessa Gordon Jason R. B. Dyck **«Improvements in skeletal muscle strength and cardiac function induced by resveratrol during exercise training contribute to enhanced exercise performance in rats»** The Journal of Physiology (2012) http://onlinelibrary.wiley.com/doi/10.1113/jphysiol.2012.230490/abstract

70 Dr Elizabeth Blackburn and Elissa Epel, *The Telomere Effect*. Grand central Publishing (2017)

71 Sung MM, Byrne NJ, Robertson IM, Kim TT, Samokhvalov V, Levasseur J, Soltys CL, Fung D, Tyreman N, Denou E, Jones KE, Seubert JM, Schertzer JD, Dyck JR: **«Resveratrol improves exercise performance and skeletal muscle oxidative capacity in heart failure».** American Journal of Physiology. Heart and Circulatory Physiology (2016) https://www.ncbi.nlm.nih.gov/pubmed/28159807.

72 David Swenson, *Ashtanga Yoga*, www.ashtanga.net.

73 Amy Cuddy, "Your Body Language May Shape Who You Are" [video], TEDGlobal (2012), https://www.ted.com/talks/amy_cuddy_your_body_language_shapes_who_you_are?

74 To learn more about the J-shaped curve visit http://www.wineanorak.com/healj.htm.

75 The French paradox, coined by Serge Renaud from Bordeaux University, was used by an American, Professor George Riley Kernodle in his book *Theatre in History* and was the subject of a documentary on the CBS programme *60 Minutes* in the 1990s. See the news item here: https://youtu.be/rMNG0zbZlmE.

76 A published study in the *Journal of American College of Cardiology* analysed the lifestyle habits and health outcomes of nearly 70,000 women over a twenty-year period.

77 Imke Janssen, Alan L. Landay, Kristine Ruppert, Lynda H. Powell, "Moderate Wine Consumption Is Associated with Lower Hemostatic and Inflammatory Risk Factors over 8 years: The Study of Women's Health across the Nation (SWAN)", *PMC: US National Library of Medicine*, 12/6 (2014), doi: 10.3233./NUA-130034, https://www.ncbi.nlm.nih.gov/pmc/articles/PMC4334149/.

78 Stefania Dragoni, Jennifer Gee, Richard Bennett, Massimo Valoti and Giampietro Sgaragli «Red wine alcohol promotes quercetin absorption and directs its metabolism towards isorhamnetin and tamarixetin in rat intestine *in vitro»* British Journal of Pharmacology (2006)* http://www.ncbi.nlm.nih.gov/pmc/articles/PMC1760706.

79 S Agewall, S Wright, R.N Doughty, G.A Whalley, M Duxbury and N Sharpe»**Does a glass of red wine improve endothelial function?**» *European Heart Journal*, 2000

80 Ruf et al. (1995); Goldberg et al. (2003). The presence of alcohol in red wine might improve flavonoid availability by increasing its intestinal absorption or by delaying its excretion. Frankel and colleagues reported in *The Lancet* in 1993 that red wine polyphenols (resveratrol and procyanidins) inhibit LDL oxidation and prevent against cholesterol, blood clotting, and inflammation independent of any action of alcohol.

81 Elizabeth Mostofsky of the Harvard School of Public Health analysed twenty-three studies of nearly 30,000 participants over twenty-eight years.

82 Mladen Boban, Creina Stockley, Pierre-Louis Teissedre, Patrizia Restani, Ursula Fradera, Claudia Stein-Hammer and Jean-Claude Ruf «Drinking pattern of wine and effects on human health: why should we drink moderately and with meals?» food anf Function '(2016) http://pubs.rsc.org/-/content/articlepdf/2016/fo/c6fo00218h.

*   Ibid

Lightning Source UK Ltd.
Milton Keynes UK
UKHW041038050120
356372UK00001B/114/P